Here is what patien[illegible]

Who Stole My Ovaries?

Newly married at age 40, I wanted to start my family soon after the reception. I followed Jane's nutrition advice, threw out my plastic stuff, and reduced stress in my life. After three months of working with Jane, I conceived my son naturally, and then at age 46, my daughter. My children and I are very healthy, but I have continued to follow her advice because reproductive health and general health go hand in hand.

~ **Sasha D.**, mother, dancer, teacher

My husband and I were so impressed with Jane's knowledge, research-based advice, and her ability to help us stay calm and positive. I am thrilled that so many other families will now get the benefit of her expertise by reading this book. We will be forever grateful to her for our family of four.

~ **Katie G.**

Infertility was not something I grew up knowing about or even learned about in nursing school. We grow up believing becoming pregnant is easy, and when we find it is not, a piece of our hope fades. Jane's holistic approach to care helped me get through the tough decisions we had to make along the way to finally having our beautiful daughter. Our frank conversations on how not to lose my identity to infertility were priceless. I feel like we were talking together again when I read her book.

~ K.S. MSN, RN, AOCNS

Without Jane's help, I would not have Lucy and Connor. In her book, she answers important questions that I had before and after trying to have a baby.

~Jillian L.

As a board-certified reproductive endocrinology and infertility specialist, I often refer patients to Jane for her holistic approach to patient care and fertility. I so appreciate her attention to important health topics such as sleep, nutrition, and relationships. Her patients tell me it feels nice to have someone like Jane on their 'team.' With this well-written, easy-to-read book, individuals can experience the true support Jane offers in personalized visits. She starts each section with a discussion over 'tea' and provides rational, well-researched data and information meant to provide support to patients during what can be a very difficult fertility journey.

~Dr. Katherine Schoyer, MD, Reproductive
Endocrinology and Infertility Specialist

I sought Jane's treatment for hormonal issues and found substantial relief. As a physician, I appreciated Jane's knowledge and expertise, always offering additional references and literature in support of her therapies.

~A. Adler, MD, MPH

In our world of complex medical solutions, Jane provides a useful and common-sense approach to conception.

~AH, father

Who Stole My Ovaries?

JANE GLEESON, RN, L.Ac.

Who Stole My Ovaries?
Enhancing Health to Improve Fertility
Recalibrating after Infertility, IVF, Pregnancy, and Miscarriages
Your Important Questions Answered

Please address all requests and permissions to:
WhoStoleMyOvaries@gmail.com.

LCCN: In Process

ISBNs:
978-1-7377381-0-7 (print)
978-1-7377381-1-4 (eBook)

Printed in the United States of America

The information in this book is not intended to take the place of the care and advice of your physician or healthcare provider.

About the cover:

The teapot was made by my friend Linda Wervey Vitamvas, who was a labor and delivery nurse for 25 years before earning an MFA in ceramics. The pot represents the uterus, and the handle and spout are fallopian tubes with an ovary at each end. The designs in the bottom of the teacups depict an egg being fertilized by a sperm and the cell division that follows. Many of her early art pieces are influenced by her years in healthcare. You can see how her work has evolved at lindavitamvas.com.

Other art credits:

Blue Tea Cup painting by Rob Gleeson
Blue and Pink Birdhouse by Summer K.
River Print image by Barb Manger
Crane Mobile by Elsa R. Photo by Neil Jaehnert.
All other photos by Jane Gleeson.

Design credits:
Photo layout by Jeanne Mueller of RedKnows, LLC
Book layout by 1106 Design

This book is dedicated to my sister Judy, a highly skilled and eccentric nurse who helped bring many babies into this world.

And to my patients, who taught me about perseverance and resilience.

Acknowledgments

I WOULD LIKE TO THANK MY HUSBAND, BOB, who encouraged me to write this book. Although he often refers to me as a "witch doctor," he is my biggest supporter and soulmate.

Elizabeth, Megan, and Rob. What can I say? Without you, I would not have known the joy and pain of motherhood. And which clothes to banish from my closet.

Thank you, Summer K., for the lovely birdhouse you painted and for your art direction on the frog photo. Thank you, Elsa R., for your crane mobile, which was the perfect image for the last section of this book. Quinn, your lighting suggestions for the cosmic egg "made" that photo. Ada, thank you for your data-entry help and for inspiring me to get this book done so that I could spend more time with you! Sister-in-law Barbara, your encouragement and books on writing that you shared were really helpful.

Thank you to my wonderful women friends who had to listen to me talk about this book for a long time.

And last but not least, I would like to thank Dr. Spencer Silver, the 3M chemist who invented the glue that resulted in stickie notes. My computer was indispensable, but I could not have stayed on track without the little squares of colored paper.

The symbol below and at the end of every section is a treskele. This triple spiral originated in the Celtic culture 6,500 years ago. Although its meaning is is interpreted in different ways, it is commonly thought to represent mental and spiritual growth through motion, action, cycles, and progress.

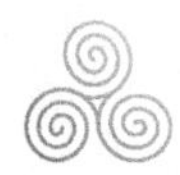

Table of Contents

Introduction

I WROTE THIS BOOK FOR MY PATIENTS and for all of you who have faced challenges as you tried to start or build your family—challenges that may have left you feeling deficient and depressed at times. My goal is to help you Renourish and Refocus as you regroup and plan your next steps.

The title, "Who Stole My Ovaries?" is meant to symbolize the frustration, disappointment, physical drain, and hormonal imbalance that accompanies fertility challenges. I hope that, after reading this book, you will feel emotionally and physically recharged and ready to forge on—symbolically, *getting your ovaries back.*

Much of the focus of this book is on a woman's experience because she is usually the one having procedures, taking hormones, needing to "get" pregnant, and "carrying" a baby, even if a male factor is involved. However, men experience the drain and stress from fertility challenges and contribute half of a baby's genes, so the information about stress reduction, nutrition, and endocrine disruptors is for them as well.

You probably assumed that, when you finished your formal education, got a good job, met your soulmate or made the decision to be a single parent, the transition from wanting to start a family and having one would be seamless. You had every right to assume that. God, Creative Intelligence, Mother Nature, or whomever you believe in designed us to procreate and wants us to do just that. Beautiful and smart babies are born every day. You also had a right to expect that you would not necessarily suffer a pregnancy loss, since most pregnancies result in happy, healthy babies.

When fertility challenges became apparent or pregnancy loss happened, you looked for answers and help. Those answers may have included being told you are not ovulating, your eggs are too old, you don't have enough sperm, your tubes are blocked, etc. Metaphorically speaking, someone stole your ovaries and sperm, and along with them, your dream of having a baby. Bad and unexpected news about your fertility may have left you drained emotionally and spiritually. The medical interventions you experienced in an effort to stay on the path to parenthood may have left you drained physically and financially. After unsuccessful IVFs and miscarriages, you may feel depressed, deficient, dejected. There are not enough "De" words in the English language to describe how one feels when your pregnancy test is negative or you have lost a baby. After trying so hard and suffering so much, you might find yourself to be a different person from the one you were before you tried to conceive. Of course, your experiences may have made you stronger, as an individual or a couple, and you need to build on those strengths. Whether you will be continuing to try to start a family or don't know what your next steps will be, this book will be helpful.

My goal in writing this book is to help you change the "De" words in your life to "Re" words. The themes of this book are Recovering, Rebuilding, Renourishing, Refreshening, and Refocusing. Your future steps for recovery will be more steady and fruitful if you have a plan.

I have noticed that my patients who have a plan for their next steps—instead of free-floating—tend to heal faster after a miscarriage or unsuccessful IVF. Your plan may include another round of IVF, taking a break from trying, continuing to try to conceive naturally, pursuing adoption, or getting a fresh look at your fertility care. Even if you change your plan, having one will help reduce your anxiety and anchor you. Our conversation will be about ways to achieve health, peace, and balance so that you are in the best place possible as you take your next steps.

This book is about your questions

One of the most rewarding parts of my practice is listening to patients and answering their questions. I feel badly when patients say, "I'm sorry that I have so many questions." I love answering questions and quite prefer it to inserting needles. I love having conversations with my patients about their pets, jobs, hopes, fears, and what they will be doing on the weekend. This tells me more about them than their lab values or their age. The questions and case histories are from real patients, but I have changed their names and some personal details to protect their privacy.

My desire to write this book came from seeing how depleting infertility struggles can be, but the selection of topics has come from my patients' questions. The answers to different patients asking the same question might differ, because no two people will have walked the exact same path. My patients may have the same Western diagnoses, but their health history, lifestyle, spirit, and steps they have already taken are unique to each of them.

I wanted this book to feel like a conversation over a cup of tea, based on what you want to know, and what I know has helped my patients over the past 20 years.

Who I am and how I hope to help you

As an RN and acupuncturist, I have specialized in women's health for the past 25 years. I have cared for hundreds of women at all stages of trying to get pregnant and those who experienced successful pregnancies. I have had hundreds of difficult conversations with women who were suffering after a miscarriage and unsuccessful IVFs. This book includes important questions from those conversations.

My healthcare career started at the College of St. Teresa (all women back then) and the Mayo Clinic (mostly men back then) decades ago. I earned a master's degree in Medical-Surgical Nursing at Emory University, where I focused on the care of neurosurgical patients. I have been a psychiatric nurse, a sexual-assault-treatment nurse, a wellness nurse, a school nurse, and a nursing instructor. I supervised teen contraceptive clinics for Planned Parenthood, where I spent time with young women who were devastated when I told them that their pregnancy test was positive. I now spend time with people who are devastated when their test is negative. While I have good credentials and experience, it is my strong desire to learn from my patients and my good listening skills that have led to my success as a health practitioner. I don't always have a solution for some of the complicated problems that a person brings to me, but being a good listener spares one "from the burden of having to give advice." When people talk with a good listener, they often identify their own solutions.

After a detour to make children and art, I returned to health-care. But I wanted to bring a fresh perspective to my work and new tools to help people. That led me to the study of Traditional Chinese Medicine, where I learned about acupuncture, herbs, Tai Chi, Qi Gong, and other ancient healing tools. My education culminated in an internship in China at the Guangzhou Hospital of Traditional Chinese Medicine. My approach to fertility and women's health combines Western and Eastern knowledge and incorporates acupuncture, nutrition education, lifestyle coaching, and stress reduction.

My own fertility journey was so long ago that I barely remember it. My first two children were conceived easily and naturally when I was in my late 20s. But at an "advanced maternal age," I decided that I *really* wanted a third child. This scared the hell out of my husband, who was at an "advanced paternal age." I once heard a doctor say, "You can't talk a woman out of wanting to have a baby." That was an understatement. So, with some help from Western Medicine (a urologist), my third child was born when his sisters were 12 and 13 years old. A second trimester miscarriage before he was conceived did not deter me from continuing to try. My son is now 30 something, and I found out recently that he had always assumed he was an unplanned, "oops baby" because he was so much younger than his siblings. Needless to say, I am all in favor of sharing a child's birth story as early as possible. While I can relate to the strong desire to have a baby as well as the deep sadness of miscarriage, no two people walk the same path and experience things in the same way. Which is why I want to get to your questions and start our conversation. You can start asking questions, right here in the introduction section.

I have already read so many books. Will I learn anything new? You are right to ask this question. By the time couples or individuals come to me for treatment, they have already read lots of books and checked out dozens of websites, articles, chatrooms, and products online.

You probably have listened to a lot of advice (often unsolicited) from many friends and relatives. Because you have been subjected to this information overload, and you already know a lot, my goal is to tweak your body of knowledge as well as simplify and clarify the most important health information.

I often suggest that patients ease up on researching everything related to fertility. I advise them to eat well, sleep well, exercise, and choose happiness. But I know the journey and the solution are not always that simple.

This book is not a comprehensive text on how to conceive or the process of IVF or the Traditional Chinese Medicine approach to fertility. There are some good books about these topics, including *It Starts with the Egg*, by Rebecca Fett, and *Taking Charge of Your Fertility*, by Toni Wechsler. *The Infertility Cure*, by Randine Lewis, is a great source of information on Traditional Chinese Medicine and fertility.

My intent is to encapsulate, highlight, and summarize the most important health information you may have learned but may now need to review in order to recalibrate, recover, reassess, re-envision, or whatever other "Re" word might be a good goal for you.

I wish that I could give you the answer to the question of why you have had to struggle to conceive or have suffered pregnancy loss. Or why your ovaries and dreams may have been diminished. But I cannot. There is no answer for that. Although there may be a "bio-medical" answer for miscarriage, such as genetic issues, there is no answer to why it happened to *you*. I do not necessarily believe that things happen in our lives for a reason. But I do believe we can bring meaning to the challenges or tragedies in our life by learning from them and choosing a course of action that helps us grow and thrive.

My hope for you is that, with some advice, guidance, and new tools, you will recover from what has been a very challenging time in your life.

I believe that tea will help with the goals of our conversation because of its spirit-settling, refreshing, and rejuvenating abilities. To that end, I have paired a tea with each section of the book. Tea has been used throughout history for health and healing, and represents harmony and peace. I love a chapter in a book by the British Drs. Steptoe and Roberts (*A Matter of Life*), who performed the first successful IVF. Their goal, which they started working on shortly after World War II, had been to help women whose fallopian tubes were blocked. After decades of setbacks, no funding, and using an old linen closet for a lab, they perfected oocyte retrieval and fertilization techniques that resulted in the birth of Louise Brown in 1978. Frequent peer criticism for trying "to play God" and being "booed" at medical conferences did not deter them along the way. When they dealt with setbacks, like three or four months with no positive pregnancy tests, they described how they would sit down with their research nurse, have a cup of tea, and talk about what may have gone wrong and what they might do differently next time. It all sounded so civilized and so British.

I wish that I could serve you a cup of tea as we converse, as I often do with patients in my office.

The patients whose stories I share are real. I have changed their names and some details to protect their privacy, but you will recognize their struggles.

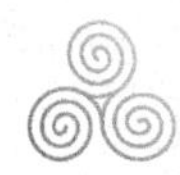

Restoring Your Spirit

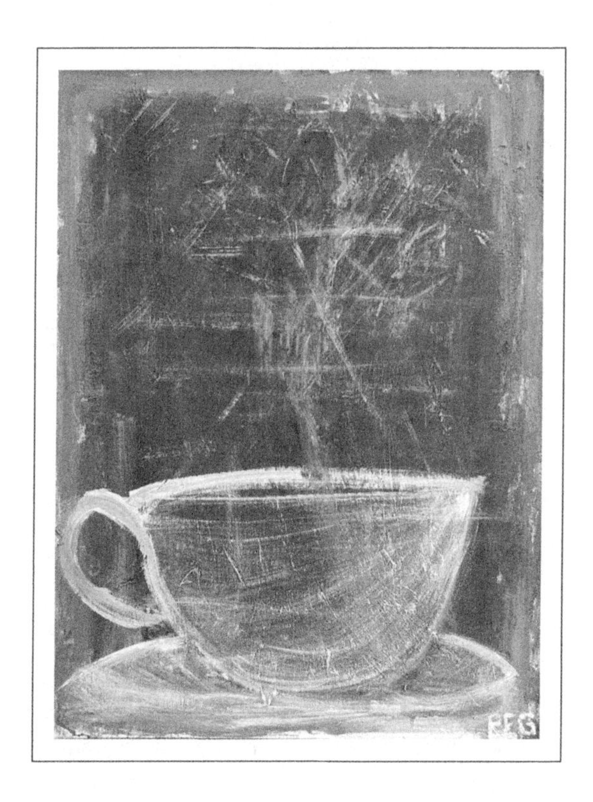

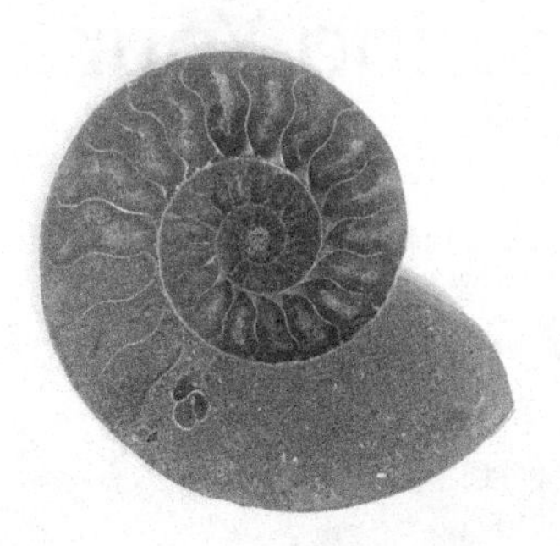

This shell known as a chambered nautilus is the outer body of a squishy sea creature who is in the same genetic clan as snails, slugs, mussels, and octopuses. The shell grows and develops in a precise mathematical pattern (the Fibonacci sequence) that is found in other parts of nature. This "sacred geometry" has led to its use as a symbol for growth and renewal. The textural and aesthetic difference between the soft squishy inside and hard outside is considered a metaphor for our inner spiritual life and our outer physical being.

A conversation over tea

Ginger is a leafy green plant with purplish green flowers; however, it is the gnarly root that is prized for its flavor and benefits. Technically, ginger tea would be a "tisane," not a tea, because the term "tea" is reserved for drinks made from the leaves of *camellia sinensis* plants, which include only green, black, white, pu-erh, and oolong teas. Hibiscus, ginger, lemon grass, and other fruit and flower teas are also tisanes. They are all enjoyable and have health benefits, so most people just refer to them as "teas."

The compounds in ginger have proven benefits for the relief of the nausea caused by pregnancy, chemotherapy, and motion. Research shows that ginger also has anti-inflammatory, antiviral, and anti-bacterial properties. Ginger tea can be made from dried ginger or by steeping fresh ginger root in water, which is my preferred method.

In traditional Chinese medicine, the warmth and heat that we experience when eating ginger enhance the "Yang" energy of our bodies, which, in turn, fuels action and movement. Ginger tea has tang and kick to it, maybe just the tonic your spirit needs.

Spirit check

THE WORD "SPIRIT" comes from the Latin word *spiritus*, meaning "breath." Some people use the word "spirit" to describe how lively or upbeat a person is, as in "She was in good spirits." The religious connotation of "spirit" is often used interchangeably with the word "soul" and refers to our essence that may live on after death. For this part of our conversation, I will use the term "spirit" to mean our inner, non-physical selves, that which animates us and gives life to our bodies. This includes our mind, emotions, character, mood, and personality. In addition to these qualities, you can also think of spirit as the vibrant parts of your personality that the world sees as well as the inner person you believe that you are.

As you read this section, just think about either term, *Spirit* or *Soul*, we are essentially talking about what makes you *you*.

Restoring spirit is what I want you to ask me about first, because I believe the human spirit is more drained than the body and more diminished by the difficulties of trying to have a baby. Your spirit must be whole and balanced to move through sadness, anger, anxiety, grief, and your next steps. If your spirit is diminished, you won't feel like eating better or exercising more or doing any of the things people tell you to do to feel better and heal. But do know that it works both ways—good lifestyle habits will nudge and maybe even propel you toward a healthy spirit.

"Diminished spirit"—do you mean "depression"?

That may be one manifestation, but often my patients have told me that they just don't feel like the person they were before trying so hard to have a baby or experiencing a miscarriage. This sense of losing the sense of who you were, although a vague feeling at times, is central to *diminished spirit*. All the ups and downs, twists and turns on your journey may have made you feel like a stranger to yourself. Our conversation will be about Returning to feeling like the old you.

Let's see where you are on the spectrum. *Diminished spirit* may include some symptoms of depression, like feeling hopeless or not being able to enjoy activities that used to bring you pleasure. Another sign that your spirit is suffering might be that you feel more irritable and unloving toward friends or perhaps with a partner who has been nothing but supportive. And then comes the guilt for being this way. Your sleep quality may be impacted when your spirit is suffering including trouble falling asleep, staying asleep, or both. The volleyball team that you have been on for years is no longer fun. Going out with friends does not appeal to you, especially if you think someone might be announcing a pregnancy. These are all understandable feelings, as you need to protect yourself from situations that trigger sadness, but they can be the signs of *diminished spirit*. When assessing patients from a Traditional Chinese Medicine viewpoint, a person with a low, soft voice, who looks down a lot instead of up, apologizes for asking questions, and seems tired although she sleeps eight hours, may have low "Qi" and *diminished spirit*. Therapists may use the term "mild depression" instead of *diminished spirit*. If you have signs of severe depression, such as the inability to work, eat, and sleep, or suicidal thoughts, I know you know to seek help from a mental-health professional.

If you have a relationship with God and/or believe in a higher power, your spirit/soul in the religious sense can suffer when you have not been able to have a baby after trying so hard. You may question why prayers have not been answered, why life was given to your baby and then taken away, or why some people who are not good parents have been blessed with children. Sometimes you need to set aside these unanswerable questions to replenish and heal, because continuing to ask them will keep draining you. Philosophers, ministers, priests, counselors, or friends may not have answers that satisfy you completely, but they can help you face not knowing these answers, which will move you closer to your "old self."

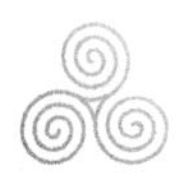

Plugging the hole in your emotional bucket

I'm not questioning my relationship with God. I just want my emotional energy back. What can I do?

FIRST, STOP THE ONGOING LOSS OF EMOTIONAL ENERGY. This is Spirit-building tool #1. If there is a hole in your bucket, you won't make much progress trying to fill it. Avoiding extremes of work and emotion can plug the hole in your emotional bucket, stem the loss of emotional energy and Restore your spirit.

The ancient Chinese Taoist philosopher Lao Tzu had some great thoughts about avoiding emotional and spiritual drain.

> Better to stop short than to fill to the brim.
> Oversharpen the blade, and the edge will soon blunt.
> Amass a store of gold and jade, and no one can protect it.
> Claim wealth and titles, and disaster will follow.

Retire when the work is done.
This is the way of heaven.
He who stands on tiptoe is not steady.
He who strides cannot maintain the pace.
He who makes a show is not enlightened.
He who is self-righteous is not respected.
He who brags will not endure.
According to the followers of the Tao
These are extra food and unnecessary luggage.
They do not bring happiness.
Therefore, the followers of the Tao avoid them.[1]

The wisdom of Lao Tzu about striving also speaks to how much energy it can take to "strive" for pregnancy. Tests, procedures, bills, internet searches, medication side effects, and insurance issues all take emotional energy. In the U.S., we use the active phrase "*getting* pregnant." England, Australia, New Zealand, and other British Commonwealth countries use the gentler phrase "falling pregnant" to describe a new pregnancy. An obstetrical textbook or article will read, "After three rounds of Clomid, the patient fell pregnant." The French phrase for conceiving is *tomber enceinte*, or "to fall pregnant." I like the imagery of *falling pregnant* rather than *getting pregnant*. It evokes the thought that one can control only so much of the mysterious process of conception. Perfectly timed intercourse and a perfect embryo transplanted into a plush lining does not result in a pregnancy most of the time.

1 Lao Tzu, *Tao Te Ching*, translation by Feng, G. and English, J. 1997

Although it is annoying when well-meaning people tell you to "just relax" and "it" will happen, letting go and letting yourself "fall" can be a soothing tonic for the Spirit. In practical terms, switching your frame of mind from "*getting* pregnant" to "*falling* pregnant" can involve revisiting natural conception if that is a viable option. Or if you have been trying to conceive naturally, consider taking a break from ovulation predictor kits and phone-based apps and just enjoy intercourse on a regular basis.

I see how hard my patients have pushed themselves to do everything right, working more hours to afford care and putting on a "happy face" for friends and family. I often talk with teachers who have experienced miscarriage and infertility, and I often feel the need to remind them that it is okay to tell your principal that you just don't want to stay after school to coach the middle-school track team. I have encouraged night-shift nurses to keep requesting day shifts because of their need for better quality of sleep; there is evidence that night-shift work may be associated with lower fertility. When you advocate for yourself, you are not being selfish or difficult—you are helping your spirit heal. You are putting your oxygen mask on first before trying to assist others.

After you have tended to your own needs, helping others can lead to spiritual growth, happiness, and a "Helpers' High."[2] Research shows that the rush of good feelings when helping others and being generous is accompanied by increased dopamine activity, which is associated with the reward system in the brain. People who volunteer have 44% lower death rates, even when the

2 Luks, A. and Payne, P. *The Healing Power of Doing Good*, iUniverse, 2001

data is adjusted for different health histories and lifestyle factors. "This is a stronger effect than exercising four times a week or going to church; it means that volunteering is nearly as beneficial to our health as quitting smoking."[3]

Remember, if you do not have the energy at this time to volunteer, or if you have not found a meaningful opportunity, just being kind to the people you come in contact with counts. Being a more courteous driver, letting a person go ahead of you in the grocery-store line, or smiling at a person you pass in the street can help restore your spirit.

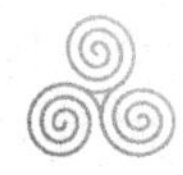

3 Christine L. Carter, "What We Get When We Give," *Psychology Today*, Feb. 18, 2010

Nurturing your positivity

MANY WOMEN ARE HEALTHY, EAT WELL, EXERCISE, meditate, have IUIs, IVFs, etc. and still do not fall pregnant. So many things need to be lined up biologically and timed perfectly for conception to occur, it is amazing that anyone gets pregnant. But women do conceive on a statistically predictable basis, so being positive is absolutely warranted. When my patients tell me that they plan to keep their expectations low so that they are not sad if a pregnancy test is negative, I guarantee them that they will feel badly if their test is negative no matter how low they set their expectations. So why not stay positive and hopeful, and enjoy those feelings for as long in a cycle as possible?

I wake up feeling positive and energized, and then a baby-shower invitation comes in the mail, and I start thinking of excuses for not attending. I'm a really bad friend, right?

You are not a bad friend! Not wanting to sit in a circle and pass booties around is a sign of *diminished spirit*, not of being a bad friend. Showers may have been fun when you rightfully thought your turn was coming.

If going to baby showers, "sprinkles," for second babies, or gender-reveal parties makes you feel sad and negative, it is okay to protect yourself and not attend. If the mother-to-be is a dear friend or treasured relative, perhaps consider sharing the true reason it would be hard for you to attend, and arrange to celebrate with them one on one. A good friend will empathize with your feelings. If you are not close to the mother-to-be, simply saying you have a scheduling conflict is okay. While this may seem selfish, protecting yourself is not selfish. You are avoiding emotional drain, plugging those holes in the bucket. I loved the response that a two-mom couple shared with me about being invited to gender-reveal parties. They wanted to say to their friends (but didn't), "Why don't you just wait until your child is about 12 and then have the party?" Too funny.

That said, I want to tell you about the benefits of not closing yourself off too much. Sarah was a skilled physical therapist and patient of mine who easily conceived twice, but, sadly, both pregnancies ended in miscarriage. She sought acupuncture treatment because she was having difficulty conceiving as she tried for a third pregnancy. She ruminated about the possibility she would never conceive again or continue to suffer miscarriages if she did. Understandably scared and depressed, her slow-burning anger was consuming her. In the ancient Eastern point of view, anger "stagnates" the body energy known as Qi and keeps it from flowing. When Qi doesn't flow, blood doesn't flow, because Qi moves the blood. When blood doesn't flow, organ systems are undernourished, including ovaries and uterus, and this does not bode well for fertility. She came to her appointment one day and said, in a very angry way, "My best friend in Chicago just emailed me that she had her baby last night. I emailed back and said, "I hope you don't take offense, but I just can't come to see you right now. It would be just too hard for me." She had emphasized the "too hard for me" and did not express happiness for her best friend's life-changing event. I gently reminded her that having a best friend is a wonderful gift from the Universe, and she should consider what it might feel like to have one of the most wonderful events of your life happen—the birth of your child—and then have your best friend choose not to share your joy. It is fine to be absent from a group event, like a shower, but probably detrimental to spirit if you damage a best-friend relationship. A few weeks later, she returned to say that she had traveled to Chicago to visit her friend and that the visit was positive and enjoyable. She had unlocked and released her anger and now felt more positive after her enjoyable visit. A few months later, she conceived and had a healthy baby girl, followed by another a few years later. The ancients would say she unlocked her mind-heart-womb connection and energy. My point is that there is a big difference between draining your spirit at baby showers, where there will be plenty of other people to "ooh" and "aah" over the breast pumps, and sharing the joy of birth with a dear friend, which can be spiritually uplifting.

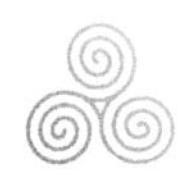

Thoughts really matter—the placebo and nocebo effect

YOU HAVE HEARD OF THE PLACEBO EFFECT, in which just hearing and trusting that a treatment or medication will work results in symptom relief. Its contribution to healing is so significant and pervasive that scientists must account for it when evaluating the results of treatments. Placebo effects have accounted for healing in everything from psoriasis and torn knee ligaments, where "sham" surgery relieved symptoms as well as "real" surgery.[4]

Placebo effects are essentially a form of positive thinking that the body responds to by tapping into the complicated and undeniable connection between the mind and the body. In Western medicine, we acknowledge that the mind can affect the body, and the body can affect the mind, but in Eastern Medicine,

4 Moseley, JB, "A controlled trial of arthroscopic surgery for osteoarthritis of the knee," July 11, 2002, *N Engl J Med* 2002; 347:81-88

mind and body are believed to be one entity. Dr. Andrew Weil's belief that "All healing starts in the mind" is a powerful thought.

I often wondered about the possibility of placebo effect and my patient Denise, who came to me at age 44. She had been trying to conceive for more than 10 years and chose not to do IVF for religious reasons. Natural conception was her only option, and she came for acupuncture treatment as part of doing everything she could to enhance her fertility. After three months of treatment and some dietary changes, Denise fell pregnant but, unfortunately, miscarried. She was so convinced that acupuncture was the reason she conceived for the first time after a decade of trying that she came right back into treatment after the miscarriage. In just a few months, she was pregnant again. Given her age and the number of years she had been trying to conceive, that short amount of time to pregnancy was remarkable. Not to diminish the effectiveness of acupuncture, I did wonder whether the acupuncture had exerted a strong placebo effect that resulted in her body really stepping up and producing just the right amounts and combinations of hormones. Believing that a treatment can help you rebalance your hormones or enhance fertility is a state of mind to be nurtured and promoted.

I wish this was not true, but placebo effect has an evil twin called the nocebo effect. You must guard against this while trying to nurture your positivity. Nocebo is the opposite of the placebo effect. That is, negative thoughts about a treatment or disease process can increase the chances that someone will experience a symptom or bad side effect.

John Kelly, PhD, and Deputy Director of the Harvard Medical School's Program on Placebo Studies and Therapeutic Encounter, observed that when people are given a placebo but told they will be having certain side effects, they do, in fact, often report those side effects. MRIs of subjects' brains showed that just imagining something bad is happening does indeed "activate those portions of the brain associated with that thought, worry, pain.[5]

"In 2012, researchers from the Technical University of Munich in Germany published an in-depth review on the nocebo effect. They looked at 31 empirical studies and found that not only does the nocebo effect exist, but it's also surprisingly common. It's also causing an ethical dilemma for doctors and nurses: If they inform patients about the potential risks and negative side effects of a given treatment (radiation, chemotherapy, surgery, and medication), the patients may believe they'll experience those harmful results, which could result in a self-fulfilling prophecy. But if they *don't* tell patients the risks, they can be sued for malpractice for violating informed-consent laws. Doctors can't leave anything out, even if they fear that providing all of the scary details may hinder their patients' recovery."[6]

Many of you have told me how angry you were at your doctor, or how sad you felt when your doctor predicted your chances of conceiving or having another miscarriage, based on statistics, your age, and lab values. Your doctor was not trying to upset you with negative thoughts; he or she was following ethical guidelines that involve full disclosure of medical information.

---

5 Govender, S, "Is the Nocebo Effect Hurting Your Health?" https://www.webmd.com/balance/features/

6 *Ibid.*

But you are not a statistic, and you have every right to believe in your ability to have a baby. If you are told that your chances of conceiving or carrying a baby using your own eggs is only 1%, you must try to focus on the fact that *you* can be the one person in one hundred.

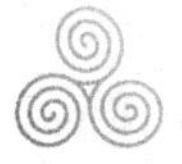

Reframing and the cup-half-full theory

IT WOULD BE RARE NOT TO HAVE A STOCKPILE of negative thoughts and beliefs about your body, your fertility, or your ability to carry a baby to term after all that you have been through.

I have talked through a lot of my negative thoughts with close friends and my therapist, but that has not kept them from coming back. How do I get out of this rut?
By not continuing to talk about them in their current form and by changing the narrative, or the "story" that led to the thoughts. While some therapists advise people to simply become comfortable with negative thoughts and not "fight" them, I am more in the reframing camp.

The decision to delay starting a family and its possible effects on current fertility challenges is a common negative thought.

Taking birth-control pills for a long time can result in amenorrhea (lack of periods) when a woman discontinues them, and this is a great setup for self-blame. If this has been a concern for you, a way to reframe this thought is to remind yourself you were being responsible by preventing an untimely pregnancy. You also made the right decision to use oral contraception, given the information available at the time regarding birth-control pills and menstrual cycles. If you delayed trying to conceive until you found the right partner, got established in your career, or earned enough to raise a child on your own, that is called *responsible decision-making.* You did not make mistakes—you made sound, responsible choices, and you deserve to be praised for that. Do not lose sight of these facts if they apply to you, reminding yourself as needed.

It's hard not to feel negative when you are told that your FSH is too high and your AMH is too low to have a good chance to conceive. My doctor said it is not likely that these numbers will change much. How do you reframe that one?

By considering that your cup is half full, not half empty.

As you probably know, follicle stimulating hormone (FSH) increases during the first part of a woman's cycle to help the egg inside the follicle grow large enough to be released and fertilized. If the FSH is higher than normal, it could be that a higher amount is needed to accomplish this growth. I have many patients of advanced maternal age with a high FSH who have regular cycles and appear to ovulate each month and do, indeed, conceive naturally. Their body is rising to the occasion by raising their level of FSH to get the job done. The cup is half full, not half empty. When a woman is clearly through menopause, her FSH declines to numbers in the normal range, as her body has figured it truly *is* done trying to conceive and that there is no need to keep increasing the FSH. I reframe the thought of a high FSH as the cup half full, not the cup half empty.

AMH (anti-Mullerian hormone) lab values can be an indicator of how many small-egg cells a woman might have in her ovaries, which is why it is used to evaluate a woman's fertility status. These smaller eggs waiting around for their chance to be chosen for ovulation spit out AMH, and a low value could indicate that there may be a low number of them. A low number of eggs does not mean that a woman is infertile. Most of my patients are not trying to have 12 children, just one or two, so if they ovulate regularly, they do, indeed, have a chance to conceive each cycle. Thinking positively with a cup-half-full rather than half-empty attitude is not a form of denial. It is being hopeful, and hope, by its nature, is something that exists despite the odds.

To be clear, though, your doctors are not misleading you or being negative when they explain that high FSH and low AMH are indicators of a fertility challenge. If you will be trying to conceive in the future, there are also some associations between FSH and AMH and the quality of eggs. Poor-quality eggs, which are in the ovaries of women of all ages, are often screened by Mother Nature and do not fertilize, or, if fertilized, result in a miscarriage. Fortunately, genetic testing and counseling can answer some (but not all) of the questions you may have about your egg quality.

The scientific method, which is the basis of modern medicine, relies on data to make predictions and conclusions. But numbers are based on group data, and you are a unique individual, not a crunched number. You are a person with every right to be the one in a better place on the bell-shaped curve.

Abigail never let anyone's cup-half-empty attitude curtail her efforts to conceive. She was a 42-year-old computer expert with an FSH of 25 (very high) and an AMH that would indicate she did not have too many "good" eggs left. IVF was, therefore, not a good option because she would not have a lot of follicles to be stimulated by the IVF medications. She and her husband, Bret, were not interested in using a donor egg, so natural conception was their only chance. Their situation was complicated by the fact that she had periods only about every 30 to 60 days and did not always have signs of ovulation prior to when her period would arrive. Michelle was about 60 pounds overweight, and her husband chewed tobacco regularly, which may have been the reason for his bad sperm report card. Abigail made a great effort to eat a more nutritious diet, although she did not lose all the weight she wanted and needed to. Bret cut way back on chewing the brown disgusting stuff. Their efforts to both improve their lifestyle habits and have intercourse more frequently to compensate for her irregular cycles paid off. Abigail conceived and delivered healthy baby Jackson at age 43. Her doctor had told her (correctly) that the chances of her conceiving naturally were "Not as low as one in a million, but pretty low." She was very happy to send him a baby photo labeled, "My one-in-a-million baby." A few years later, they were actively trying for a sibling for Jackson. They wanted their children close in age, so they chose to use a donor egg and Bret's sperm to accomplish that. I was honored when she asked me to look at the donor registry with her.

My patient Shonda never knew what her "ovarian reserve" (FSH and AMH) numbers were when she married at age 42. When she first came to me for acupuncture, she was not at all concerned about her age and had not seen a doctor. She intended to find one when she got pregnant. Her delightful, albeit naïve, attitude about her chances of conceiving were refreshing and a real lesson for me.

Although of advanced maternal age, Shonda had some great things going for her. As a professional dancer, she was very fit, ate well most but not all the time, and may have inherited nice longevity genes—her mother was 46 when Shonda was born. She conceived after about four months of nutrition counseling, stress-reduction efforts, and acupuncture treatments. Carter was safely delivered by C-section after his broad shoulders got stuck in the birth canal. Four years later, she conceived naturally again and gave birth to a healthy baby girl. Shonda was determined to have a vaginal birth after her previous C-section, and with the help of her supportive family practitioner, that is exactly what she did. I often wondered what her FSH and AMH were at age 47, but she never got them checked.

In my 20 years in practice, I have had the joy of treating many women with histories like those of Abigail and Shonda. Their stories are not anomalies, and their babies were not "miracle babies." Chances for conception are based on aggregate data, an averaging and mash-up of data from many people. You, like my patients, are more than the sum of your parts. You are a whole person with an almost-infinite number of emotional, physical, and experiential facts that apply only to you.

If you try to conceive in the future and are concerned about your age, I recommend reading an article by Jean Twenge. In the article, she sheds light on the statistics concerning fertility in women of "advanced maternal age" that is positive and enlightening.[7]

---

7 Twenge, JM, "How Long Can You Wait to Have a Baby?" *The Atlantic,* July/August 2013.

To keep a positive mindset, certain medical terms need to be reframed. Maybe you had the experience of not producing a lot of follicles when taking maximum doses of Follistim and were labeled a "non-responder." I want to help you reframe the situation and leave labels like that behind. The ovaries were designed to make only one egg per month, and two or three is rare. But ovaries can be "tricked" into making many more than that with the help of the IVF medications. When, on occasion, astounding numbers of eggs do not begin to grow during stimulation, I tell women that they are not broken or malfunctioning. A positive reframe is that your body wisdom may be trying to put the brakes on a forced process. If the ovaries could talk, they might say, "Whoa, what are you trying to do? We can grow 18 follicles, but do you really want 18 children all at once?" A woman who is labeled a "non-responder" may, indeed, have a very wise body.

Not making assumptions is key to reframing and its link to positivity. Jen had been trying to conceive naturally when she turned to the internet for answers. She was doing beautiful temperature charting, and her midcycle temperature spikes clearly indicated she was ovulating. But after three more months with no pregnancy, she came to my office, sad, negative, and with her self-diagnosis. "I never have any of that slippery, shiny, stringy mucus you are supposed to have." Yes, I told her, the mucus is an important indication of impending ovulation, but it is entirely possible that your mucus just stayed up around the cervix, where it is produced, instead of dripping down for you to see. Part of the job of the fertile mucus may be to meet and greet the sperm swimming upstream, to rehydrate them during their long journey to the fallopian tubes. Staying up near the cervix instead of flowing down may be just what was needed by her body. I have advised several of my patients who felt sad and negative about not seeing fertile mucus to ask their doctors if they see any when they are preparing to do an intrauterine insemination. Jen did so and happily reported back, "I asked her, and he said I had a ton of mucus up there!"

It would be normal to feel negative and perhaps hopeless if you don't ovulate regularly, as can be the case with polycystic ovarian syndrome (PCOS). But as long as you have eggs, you have a good chance of conceiving naturally or with the many medical interventions available.

I sometimes worry that I may be encouraging false hope when I help patients reframe their negative thoughts and think more positively about their eggs that won't come out, the cervical mucus they can't find, or their less-than-ideal FSH and AMH. I sometimes wonder if the silver lining I try to find for my patients or my lemonade-from-lemons approach is my own inability to deal with the sadness of others. But I will say it again: the nature of hope is that it involves wanting something to occur that is indeed against the odds. Whether that hope is returning to hormonal and emotional balance or conceiving, healing starts with allowing yourself to reframe negative thoughts and nurture positive thoughts.

Sure, I can tell myself that my cup is half full and purge negative thoughts from my head, but how am I supposed to handle it when people outside my head are hurling negative thoughts at me and telling me my cup is half empty?

You mean when your doctor tells you that you have a 2% chance of conceiving with your own egg "at your age"?

Yes, exactly.

Although many of my patients have felt the delivery of negative information is often lacking compassion, doctors try to move to the solutions and interventions they have to offer, rather than try to process what a patient is feeling when they hear grim news. Counselors, therapists, support groups, and dear friends can fill that need. The move to discuss solutions and possible interventions even though a patient is still reeling from bad news is a doctor's way of being hopeful and moving forward, which is what you want to do. Could some doctors be a bit more compassionate in their delivery? Of course, like the doctor who dragged out his egg catalogue at my patient's first visit after he looked at her numbers. With great enthusiasm, he related that he had seen a photo of a new donor that very morning and exclaimed, "She looks just like you!" This couple had barely heard of donor eggs and thought they were going to someone who would help them get pregnant naturally. When the husband morosely asked what would happen if they tried IVF with their own eggs anyway, the doctor replied that his money would be better spent on buying a boat if they wanted to try with their own egg. Although this doc's initial directness was never appreciated, he was an excellent physician and truly worked hard for patients who were already several years behind on their family-building plan. Many patients told me they appreciated his directness because they felt it saved them time and perceived that his goal was the same as theirs—to have them bring a baby home as soon as possible. See how I made this into a positive narrative?

While it is not productive to question the doctor's statistics or to try to prove him or her wrong, it is productive to reframe the thoughts for the purpose of staying positive and rebuilding spirit.

Some more examples for reframing thoughts:

Old thought: "The chances of conceiving at my age are only 2%."

New thought: "That means two women out of a hundred women my age will bring home a baby. I can be one of them."

Old thought: "My mother-in-law is really not respecting boundaries by asking me when we are going to start a family. We have been trying hard, but the details are none of her business."

New thought: "My mother-in-law is so eager to see me happy and have our family grow. I can probably sign her up for Tuesday and Thursday baby care when I go back to work."

Old thought: "We probably have to do IVF. What if my baby has a problem in the future because of the IVF process?"

New thought: "Although there is a higher incidence of birth defects in IVF babies as opposed to naturally conceived babies, some of the defects are mild and correctable. IVF provides an opportunity to genetically test cells to aid in choosing a healthy embryo, therefore potentially avoiding birth defects." Dr. Alan Penzias, of Boston IVF, has a positive view on this question: "Fortunately, the overwhelming majority of children born after in vitro fertilization are healthy . . . The positive impact on families who would not otherwise exist without fertility treatment is immeasurable."[8]

If you feel that your negative thoughts or those of others keep circling in your mind, try this: Make a list of those thoughts in a column, and then, in the next column, rewrite them. Be brave,

8 https://www.medpagetoday.com/obgyn/infertility/89388

creative, and possibly humorous when coming up with new thoughts for old ones. When an old thought comes to mind, summon the new one, and push the other one out. Recurrent thoughts can fade with time, but not always, so practice this strategy.

I'd love it if you shared some of your reframed thoughts with me at WhoStoleMyOvaries@gmail.com. I am always looking for good ones to suggest to patients.

We have talked about renewing spirit in the sense of mood, personality, and energy. *Spirit* defined as the *essence that may live on after death and that which encompasses a relationship with a higher power* is something that I know is important to you. Prayer, along with yoga and "playing with my cats," is a common answer to the *What do you do for stress relief?* question on my intake form. This does not surprise me because studies show that 80% of people pray and believe in a higher power.

I do not ask people if they pray or about their belief system unless they want to discuss it. But I am always happy when patients tell me they have a spiritual or religious life. In retrospective studies, meaning just asking people if they pray and comparing their health to people who have not developed a spiritual life, it is clear that spirituality is associated with better mental and physical health. *The Healing Power of Prayer,* by Dr. Harold Koening, professor of psychiatry and Director of the Duke University Center for the Study of Religion, Spirituality, and Health, is a great source of information on how spirituality, which includes faith and prayer, leads to better health outcomes.

If you practice an organized religion, it can be comforting to explore its traditions regarding fertility. In Catholicism, we have a patron saint for everything. There is a long list of historical figures who can be prayed to for fertility, including Saints Colette, Catherine, Bridgid, and Gianna.

Some of my patients struggle with their religion's dogma and negative viewpoint on IVF. Catholicism considers it immoral, and Mormons and Evangelicals discourage it on moral grounds as well. But I have consoled women by sharing my belief that Mother Nature and Creative Intelligence have been concerned for some time about how endocrine-disrupting pollutants have been working against the fertility of our species, and they thereby revealed the knowledge of assisted reproduction.

Religions have dispensed fertility advice throughout the ages, as in the Talmud, which suggests how frequently a man should have intercourse if he is trying to have children. Secular fertility-support groups like Resolve (https://resolve.org/support/find-a-support-group/) are excellent resources and many fertility clinics offer support groups. I encourage patients to consider faith-based groups if their spiritual life has a religious component. In Judaism, an organization called *Yesh Tikva* (Hebrew for "there is hope") (https://yeshtikva.org) provides tools and strategies for people trying to conceive. There is a *Tehillim for Children* program (*tehillim* is the Hebrew word for "psalms") available through WhatsApp. Volunteers of the organization recite psalms on behalf of those who have been struggling to conceive.

My work is my prayer for patients, but, on occasion, I ask the Blessed Virgin Mary (who seems to have had quite an intriguing fertility journey herself) to intervene for them if possible.

In Japan, I watched dozens of women seeking to conceive pray and place little plastic babies at the shrine of Inari Okami, a Shinto fertility goddess. As I entered the inner sanctum that protected her statue, I was undeterred by the expression on the face of the monk guarding it, which seemed to say, "You're not really going to try for a baby at your age, are you?" Had I been fluent in Japanese, I would have explained to the monk that when I travel, I like to bring home good-luck charms and chotzkies for my patients from places like this shrine. But that was way too much to type into Google Translate.

One of the best compliments I have ever received was from a patient's father who was aching to become a grandfather. When his daughter finally conceived, he introduced me at a party with an exuberant, "She did what ten years of my saying the Rosary couldn't do." While I was flattered, I believe in the tipping-point theory: We need to stack up a lot of positive stuff and action to achieve the result we want. His prayers undoubtedly helped.

A broad view of prayer includes meditation, mental intentionality, focused attention, contemplation of a divine power, or interconnectedness. If you do not have a belief system that includes a God to whom you pray (Buddhists offer prayers for the Universe, not to a God), you can still have a spiritual life that has the potential to enhance physical health and life goals.

Regaining a Sense of Calm

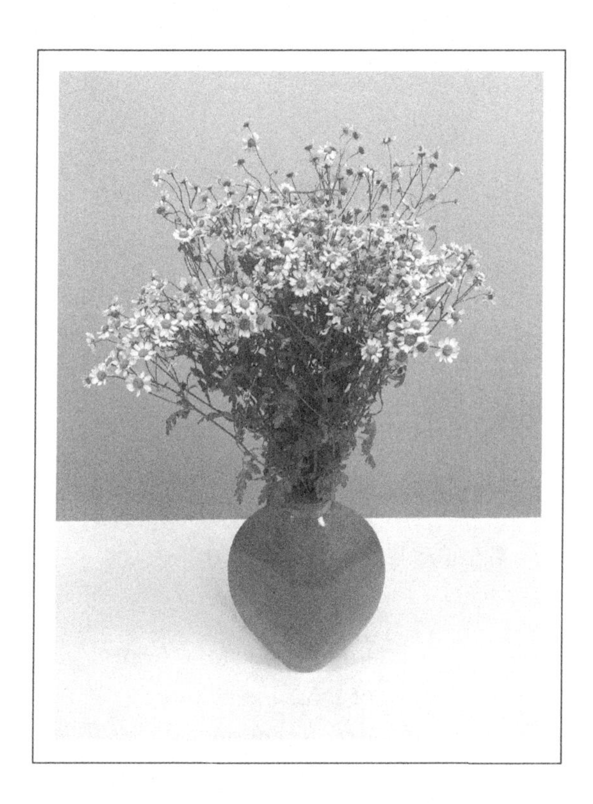

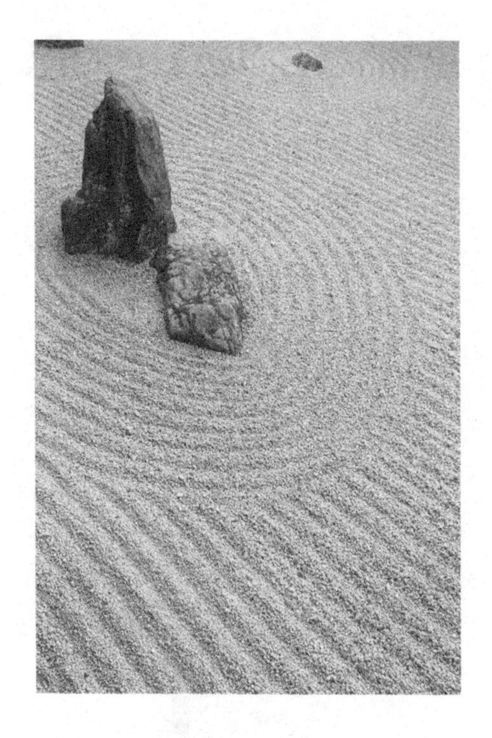

Zen Gardens come to us from
ancient Japanese culture.
They represent peace,
unadorned simplicity,
order, and a place to meditate.

A conversation over tea

Chamomile, a member of the daisy family, has been used in traditional medicine for thousands of years to calm anxiety and settle stomachs.

Enjoying two to three cups per day might be a good place to start. For anxiety reduction, I would recommend starting with a weaker tea early in the day and sipping it slowly throughout the day. If your goal is to have better-quality sleep, I would drink some closer to bedtime and make it a little stronger. You can also add honey, which has gentle sedative effects. Remember, teas are "slow food" medicine and their effects incremental.

There are some references in the literature to chamomile as a uterine "toner" and emmenagogue, which is a substance that can bring on a period or cause contractions. One study showed that concentrated capsules of chamomile induced labor in some women who were past their due date. Although the evidence is not conclusive, it is probably best not to drink a lot of strong chamomile tea if you are pregnant and to drink none at full term.

Stop stressing about stress

WHEN MY PATIENTS TELL ME that they feel stressed, they usually mean they are feeling tense, worried, nervous, and strained, rather than tranquil or calm. Stress and anxiety travel together, with stress caused by things that are happening or did happen. Anxiety is more anticipatory in nature, resulting from thinking about things that may or may not happen. Stress and anxiety reduce the joy of feeling tranquil and calm. Embracing strategies to decrease them will help you regain your sense of calm.

Jobs, relationships, and finances are frequently listed when I ask my patients about their sources of stress. Even colors and numbers become a source of stress and anxiety when people are trying to conceive. Is the line on the pee stick pink, or am I seeing things? How many follicles are growing on each ovary? How many millimeters is my uterine lining? Is my HCG level going up or down? How many weeks will it take to get a period after my miscarriage? Concerns about these numbers are rarely accompanied by a sense of calm.

I feel stressed and not very calm at times. Do you think this caused my trouble getting pregnant or my miscarriage?

Not necessarily, and I sense that you are stressing about stress. When added to other things like poor nutrition and poor-quality sleep, stress may contribute and tip the scales toward reduced fertility.

We know that hormones such as cortisol and catecholamines are released by our glands and organs during acute stress to prepare our heart and muscles for the "Fight or Flight" response. Since it is probably not a good time to get pregnant when a tiger is chasing you, Mother Nature kindly arranged for these stress hormones to block reproductive hormones and reduce non-essential functions like digestion and reproduction. The National Institutes of Health and the University of Oxford looked at amylase (a steroid and biomarker of stress) in the saliva of women trying to conceive. They found that women with the highest levels of amylase had lower fertility rates compared to women with low amylase.[9]

But the extent to which non-life-threatening sources of stress impact fertility or disrupt pregnancy is not clear. Dr. Alice Domar, a Harvard Associate Professor and founder of the Mind Body program at Boston IVF, concluded that 14 years of data does not answer the question of whether depression, stress, and anxiety cause infertility. However, her research did indicate that intervention for stress

---

9 NIH News Release, August 11, 2010. Originally published online in *Fertility and Sterility*. https://www.ncbi.nlm.nih.gov/pubmed/24664130

was associated with a much higher pregnancy rate. Women who participated in a Mind/Body stress-reduction program had a 76% pregnancy rate versus the control group, who did not participate and had a 43% pregnancy rate.[10]

My sister-in-law is a bucket of stress. She stresses out about everything, and she has four kids. How can that be if stress is so bad?

Two reasons: one is that stress may have an upside, and, two, there are levels of stress, as in everyday stress and life-threatening stress.

In her book *The Upside of Stress*, health psychologist Dr. Kelly McGonigal writes about the difference in the body's response between major stressors, like divorce or job loss, and "everyday" stress, like from bosses who micromanage or arguments with a beloved spouse. She believes that stress helps us find creative solutions, focus, and connect with others as well as increases motivation.

While everyone agrees that divorce, death of a loved one, and job loss are big stressors, individual responses to stress vary. Before working with people trying to conceive, I assumed that doctors, nurses, and high-level executives would have the highest levels of stress. That is not what I see in my practice. I have learned that tradesmen and teachers often have the highest levels of stress. Brendon was a union plumber who had to deal with deadlines on commercial installations, with big financial penalties attached to them. These were often deadlines that his bosses

10 Alice D. Domar, et al., Impact of a group Mind/Body Intervention on pregnancy rates in IVF patients. *Fertility and Sterility, In Vitro Fertilization* Vol 95 Issue 7, pp. 2269-2273, June 1, 2011

agreed to without knowledge of how long it would actually take to get the work done. The responsibility to get quality work done in an unrealistic amount of time may have been a factor contributing to his low libido. He was exhausted and worried when he got home each night.

Some of the most stressed patients I see are teachers. They work hard to prepare for parent-teacher conferences at schools in which either few parents will show up, or dozens of "helicopter parents" descend on them demanding to know why their little Einstein has not been challenged enough.

It is possible that, if your sister-in-law with the four kids stresses about things like the carpool or grocery shopping with a toddler in tow, it is a lower-level, "good type" of stress that has helped her come up with the coping strategies that Dr. McGonigal writes about.

How do I determine if my stress is at an okay level or might be harming me?

There can be physical signs of harmful stress, like high blood pressure and gastrointestinal problems, although these things can have other causes. Disrupted and poor-quality sleep is a common complaint that many of my patients attribute to stress. But it is a bit of a cycle—poor-quality sleep can affect your ability to deal with potentially stressful events, and stressful events can impact your sleep. Intervention at any part of the cycle is part of the solution.

When I meet with patients for the first time, I have a brief but effective way of helping them gauge their stress level.

I ask them to rate themselves from one to ten. A number ten is, "I need to see a therapist or counselor" or, if they already are in counseling, "I need to go more often." A number ten would also be, "I think I might be a candidate for medication." Some people rate themselves as a one or two, which I love to hear. I am sad to hear, "I am a 12 on a scale of 10." It is interesting that, if patients are coupled, a partner will often express shock and disagreement with the number given by their partner, saying things like, "Oh, no—you are much higher than that!"

I want to think about what number I would be, but can I assign a different number for stress from work, from my relationship, from trying to get pregnant and . . .

Wait, stop. No. Only one number. Although you probably can compartmentalize some of your stress, you are just one person with one mind and one body. I have acupuncture points for stress reduction, but the ancients did not leave recipes with separate points for job, marriage, and health-related issues.

I encourage people to think about all the sources and the intensity of their subjective feeling of stress and come up with one number. My assessment tool is not a scientific, validated one that a PhD in psychology would use to make a diagnosis. It is designed to have people reflect on their feelings and to help me determine how many "relaxing" acupuncture points I will use or if I will suggest professional counseling. If you assign yourself a number that sounds high to you, or you're concerned about physical symptoms that may be related to stress, sorting things through with your care provider or a good counselor is wise.

If you do not want to go to counseling or if finding the time and money to go presents another source of stress, I have some self-care strategies I would like to share with you.

If you are going to suggest meditation and yoga, I already tried those when I went through my second unsuccessful IVF. I didn't stick with the meditation, though—can you tell me about it again? I would be happy to tell you about meditation again, as well as share some other strategies you may not have tried.

Meditation comes from the healing traditions of many ancient cultures. There are many types of meditation, including Mindful Meditation, Zen meditation, Kundalini Breathing, and, of course, the online guided meditation apps like Headspace and Calm. They are all helpful, but I recommend practicing Mindful Meditation, because there are truckloads of research supporting its relaxation benefits, and there is not as much research on many other types.

Remember: the origin of the English word "spirit" is the Latin word for "breath," *spiritus*. Mindful Meditation is a breath-based meditation proven to decrease high blood pressure and anxiety and to increase cognitive function, happiness, and your sense of well-being. Dr. Herbert Benson, a Harvard cardiologist, started to look at the effects of meditation on hypertension back in the 1970s and more recently looked at evidence that meditation may be able to alter genes associated with our physiological responses to stress.[11]

In an effort to convince people to meditate, I like to explain the science of why something as simple as focusing on the breath can have such wide-ranging effects.

The big kahuna of our nervous system is the brain and spinal cord. But there are two other parts of the nervous system, called the "parasympathetic" and the "sympathetic" systems. When acute

11 https://www.sciencedaily.com/releases/2013/05/130501193204.htm

stress or fright occurs, the actions of sympathetic nerves result in an increase in muscle tension, blood pressure, heart rate, and respiratory rate, helping you get ready to fight or flee. Cortisol is released from your adrenal glands, which helps this response take place. But too much chronic dripping of cortisol or tension in our arteries can cause disease. The built-in counterbalance to this mechanism (the Yin to all of this Yang) is the parasympathetic system. When it is activated, your blood vessels will dilate, lowering your blood pressure, and your muscles will relax. Brain studies have shown that Mindful Meditation or Mindful Breathing, as it is sometimes called, activates the parasympathetic nervous system, inducing the relaxation response and decreasing the sympathetic nervous system "fight or flight" response.[12]

The essence of Mindful Meditation is focusing on the breath. Although the theories behind the therapeutic and physiologic effects of Mindful Meditation are complex, I believe it might be quite simple—we sometimes get so involved in a thought, a tense emotion, or plowing through mounds of email, that we hold our breath for fractions of a second, without even realizing it. The negative physiological effects of these momentary pauses in breathing, called "email apnea," are described by James Nestor in his book *Breath*. He calls breathing the "Missing Pillar of Health," and Mindful Meditation's benefits may indeed be that it ensures that we are not intermittently holding our breath. He posits that panic attacks (which are accompanied by many of the fight-or-flight symptoms) may have little to do emotions and more to do with a breathing problem.

---

12 Zaccaro, A., "How Breath-Control Can Change Your Life: A Systematic Review on Psycho-Physiological Correlates of Slow Breathing," *Front Hum Neuroscience* 2018;12:353

Mindful Breathing is part of a whole mindful approach to life that involves paying attention to eating, walking, driving—essentially everything we do all day long. Focusing on the breath is simply a way of staying in the present moment, which is a welcome respite for our multi-tasking minds. If you have ever seen an infant play with her foot or a toddler emptying out a drawer or cupboard, you will see mindfulness in action. Little ones are truly in the present moment, a skill and awareness we lose with age.

Can Mindful Meditation help my out-of-whack hormones?
Possibly. Researchers at UC Davis and Georgetown have shown that Mindful Meditation can lower two types of stress hormones, cortisol and ACTH. Stress hormones interact with reproductive hormones through a connection Mother Nature designed and which we call the hypothalamic-pituitary-gonadal axis. I think Mother Nature has yet to totally reveal the genius behind her design. "Out of whack" hormones are a problem you want to get on top of, as we know that estrogen and progesterone have been shown to directly affect the neurotransmitters that regulate mood, appetite, and sleep. If you have been through fertility treatment, this is probably not news to you.

What follows is my quick guide to Mindful Meditation, so that you can get started without taking a class or checking out YouTube videos. It may vary a bit from some "purists" who believe, for example, that you should not meditate while lying down because you might fall asleep. I say *Who cares* if you fall asleep, as long as you get some meditation in before you fall asleep. Mindful Meditation has been a great aid to many of my patients who struggle with getting to sleep. Of course, you will get more benefits if you meditate longer instead of falling asleep, but you are allowed to start and end where you want to.

* Sit or lie in a comfortable position with your eyes closed or in "soft focus." (Taking your glasses off can help with soft focus.)

* Breathe in through the nose and out through the nose.

* Focus on the sound of the breath if you can hear one.

* Focus on the feel of the breath in the nose.

* You can visualize your breath entering and leaving your lungs, if that keeps you focused on the breath.

* When thoughts come into your mind, observe what they are, let them go, and go back to the breath.

Start out with a goal of just 10 minutes per day. Work up to at least 20 minutes per day, as research has shown that this amount of time will result in therapeutic benefits. Do not criticize yourself for having thoughts as your mind wanders away from the thought of the breath.

I have tried breathing meditation, and the thoughts just keep coming. What am I doing wrong?
Nothing. Remember: Mindful Meditation is not about "clearing" your mind. It is not possible to clear your mind. Our minds were

designed to think thoughts and continue to do so even when we are asleep—it's called dreaming. We may not remember our dreams, but we have them through the various cycles of sleep. You can no more tell your mind to stop having thoughts than tell your heart to stop beating or your lungs to stop breathing. It is automatic and autonomic.

I believe our minds were designed to "multitask," which makes it harder to think only about the breath. Multi-tasking has been an important survival skill from the beginning of time, when a caveman had to watch the cave door for lions at the same time he was rubbing sticks together to start a fire. Multitasking is an important skill with our busy lifestyles and careers, so thoughts will still come to you as you try to focus on your breath. Recognize what the thought is about and let it float out. When I ask my patients to meditate during their acupuncture treatments, I know they are often thinking, *Jeez, it will be 5:00 when I get out of here. What should I make for dinner? Should we go out? Should we have leftovers? Should we not have dinner?* These thoughts would lead to other thoughts about *which* restaurant or *which* leftovers. The most helpful response to this is to say to yourself, *Oh, I'm thinking about dinner. I want to go back to the breath.* Do this instead of going off with the menu of options. Most of the time, when thoughts come in, they involve something that happened in our past, or something that may happen in the future. Important thoughts will come back to you after meditation, so let them go. Do not criticize or judge yourself for having thoughts—it's a normal part of the process. Just stay neutral. Going back to the breath is part of the meditation practice.

If you have difficulty staying with the breath when you meditate, try this counting technique. Take in a breath and say "one" as you exhale. Take the next inhalation, and say "two" as you exhale. In other words, don't count each inhalation, just the exhalation. Count only to 10, and then start over at "1," because it could be cumbersome to be breathing and saying to yourself, "Two thousand, five hundred and eighty-four."

What is the best time of day to meditate?
The best time to meditate is any time that is consistent. That way, you will form a habit.

If you lie in bed for a while and plan your day before jumping out of bed in the morning, I suggest doing your meditation first, and then planning your day. Your day *will* unfold—whether you lie in bed thinking about it or not. If you tend to take a while to get to sleep at night, do your meditation then. If you feel that you are falling asleep fairly soon into meditation, perhaps you might sit up in bed instead of lying down.

I pray regularly. That's like meditation, right?
Yes, there are definite similarities between prayer and meditation.

Some types of breath-based meditation with proven therapeutic effects involve breathing in for five or six seconds and breathing out for five or six seconds. This would slow your respiratory rate to about six breaths per minute rather than the usual 14 to 20. Interestingly, Buddhist, Taoist, Native American, Hindu, and many other cultures have developed chants and prayers that involve this five- or six-second breathing cycle when recited. According to a study done at the University of Pavia, the Hail Mary's of the Catholic rosary fall into this pattern.

Prayer can help you heal because it is part of cultivating spirituality, which helps you feel calmer and less stressed.

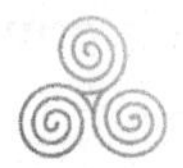

Play

A WORD OFTEN USED INTERCHANGEABLY with "play" is *recreate* or *recreation*. Re-creating parts of your spirit through play is a strategy worth considering.

We are hardwired for play, and we may have a "biologically programmed need for play," according to Dr. Stuart Brown.[13] It's how kittens, puppies, and humans learn about the world. For humans, it remains an important activity all through life. Play shares some characteristics with meditation, as we are mostly in the moment when we play. Watch a child shut the world out and focus as they color, move toy cars around, or search for the best place for hide-and-seek. Play gives us a built-in opportunity for socialization, creativity, and physical exercise.

---

13 Brown, Stuart *Play: How it Shapes the Brain, Opens the Imagination, and Invigorates the Soul*. Avery Publishing Group, 2009, page 127.

I don't feel very playful. I have had so many disappointments. What things count as "play"?

Play can be organized, as in playing on a volleyball team, or more expansive and spontaneous.

I agree with Dr. Brown that "Defining play has always seemed to me like explaining a joke—analyzing it takes the joy out of it." Nonetheless, he wrote a whole book describing and explaining the importance of play. Play can sometimes seem to be purposeless, and in our purpose-driven lives, sometimes a break from goals and purpose can be refreshing. "Lack of play . . . can be like malnutrition . . . a health risk to mind and body."[14]

Striving so hard to have a baby can put you at risk for not finding the time to play. And even if you have the time, you may often not be in the mood to play. You have pictured yourself at play with your baby, and when that is not happening, play just does not seem appealing. But play can help you heal and is probably the most fun of all the strategies we will talk about.

Look at what you were doing for fun or play before your schedule filled up with doctor's appointments, blood draws, and ultrasounds. Did you paint, hike, play cards with a group? Getting back in touch with your inner kid is the goal here. Did you like Play-Doh? Maybe look into a ceramics course. In workshops given by my friend Linda (the cover artist), I have made some oddly fun objects that emerged by just playing with a lump of clay. If you were a tree climber, maybe now is the time to explore rock-climbing walls.

My patient Kelly never left organized play behind as she went through a series of unsuccessful IUIs and two IVFs. She and her

---

14 Brown, *op. cit.*, page 215

husband Jake were in a volleyball league that was vital to her sense of well-being and helped get her through the days when the pregnancy tests that followed her embryo transfers were all negative. I was concerned about her jumping up to spike the ball at a time when she was asking her ovaries to grow multiple eggs. I asked her to quit the team for a while. She explained that having fun with her teammates meant too much to her to quit, especially at this challenging time in her life. Her first IVF transfer failed, but her second one resulted in her beautiful, healthy son. I see now that playing volleyball was pure fun for her. It involved movement, socialization, and a nice respite from the stress of trying to have a baby. Strive to keep team sports non-competitive, though, because play is intrinsically lighthearted and not goal driven. "Play should bring you a significant amount of joy without offering a specific result . . . That means taking a bike ride because it's fun, not because you are trying to lose five pounds" advises Jeff Harry, positive psychology coach.[15]

It is no coincidence that corporations often gather their stressed-out employees for a team-building, fun experience that involves playing some kind of sport. I recently watched a group of bank employees taking their first curling lesson at the Petit Ice Arena. Curling is much harder than it looks, and you could tell that just stepping on the ice was scary for some of the people. Their curling teacher explained to me, "People are unsure at first, and then you can just see them relax after a while and have fun." Fun is the essential element of play. Consider something new to you, but if pushing a heavy rock around on ice does not

---

15 Wong, Kristin "How to Add More Play to Your Grown-Up Life," *New York Times*, Aug 14, 2020.

sound like fun, complete this sentence, "I have always wanted to try ______."

Former bouncer, tango dancer, and spiritual leader Pope Francis (yes, the current Pope) shares his secret to happiness: "Slow down. Take time off. Live and let live. Don't keep negative feelings bottled up. Enjoy art. Enjoy books. Play."[16]

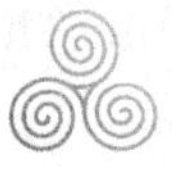

16 Egan, Timothy, *Pilgrimage to Eternity: From Canterbury to Rome in Search of Faith* 2019.

Start a huge, foolish project

"START A HUGE, FOOLISH PROJECT—it doesn't matter what people think of you" is a quote often attributed to Rumi, a 13th-century Persian philosopher.

Starting a huge, foolish project sounds like an invitation to play and tap into your creativity. I struggled with my vision of what I wanted to share with you and how to make it into a cohesive book. I had writer's block, and I had not even started to write. But thinking of this book as my huge, foolish project got me started and kept me going. This book is not foolish, because I wanted to share everything that might help you. Your foolish project can be made with paper, paint, crayons, clay, chalk, wood, bricks, flowers, or on an iPad. Hobbies, like scrapbooking or photography, are a form of play that can morph into a huge project.

Alli was a 44-year-old yoga instructor when she met and married Dan, who was about 15 years younger. They had one successful

IVF but suffered a miscarriage, after which they determined that conceiving naturally was their best option, given her age and their finances. She was always healthy, but after the failed IVF, they took things up a notch in terms of healthy eating and exercise. There is a lot of pressure on women older than 40 when they try to conceive, and it can be even more intense when a woman's partner is younger. The assumption is that any problems with conceiving are most likely due to the woman, and, of course, we know that this is not always true. Dan was a tree doctor and could often be found up in trees injecting toxic chemicals to save them from disease. The potential effect of the chemicals on his sperm quality did concern the three of us, but he did the best he could by wearing protective clothing and showering and washing his clothes immediately after work. Dan and Alli rotated weekly acupuncture treatments, which were aimed at increasing blood flow to both of their reproductive organs. Better blood flow to organs leads to better function of organs.

Although Alli had her share of teary days when her period would start, she was by nature a very positive and upbeat person. In addition to seeing her smiling face every other week, I really looked forward to seeing the projects she would work on in my waiting room. She would sit and make these funny, funky little dolls out of scraps of interesting cloth. She also made a line of tiny purses, adorned with buttons, bows, and beads. Talk about a foolish project—who needs tiny purses that couldn't even fit a credit card? But it was so obvious they were made with love and fun. She and Dan conceived about eight months into treatment, and she had a healthy baby boy at age 46. I am convinced that her creative sewing projects helped calm her and carry her through the stressful and down times during those months.

I have lots of foolish projects all over my house and basement. Not good, right?

Basements are the museum of hobbies. If your projects are creating clutter, adding another project is probably not a good calming, de-stressing activity for you.

Clutter is associated with higher levels of stress, hence the appeal of Marie Kondo's "Life Changing" decluttering techniques. But as Ms. Kondo wisely points out, the burst of energy you get from getting rid of crap won't last if you don't address foundational reasons for stress.

What I do recommend is to get rid of the trappings of what you have been through. They are reminders of where you have been but not where you need to go. Throw out expired supplements, properly dispose of needle containers and medications you won't be using, and remove the fertility-related books you have accumulated at your bedside. You can always get those things back if you need them.

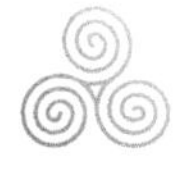

Write

I don't see myself making stuff with a glue gun or climbing up a rock wall. I like to write. Can writing help my stress and spirit?

ABSOLUTELY. Writing poems and short stories is a great creative outlet. Writing down thoughts, feelings, and observations, referred to as "journaling," improves mood and lowers anxiety. Journaling will not take away your painful longing for a baby, but it can reduce depressive symptoms while going through IVF.[17]

There is some overlap between creative writing and journaling, as sometimes a poem is inspired by a heartfelt journal entry. Many of you have been through so much trying to have a baby that, if you wrote it all down, you would have a compelling book.

Psychologist and pioneer in the field of writing therapy James Pennebaker discovered that students who were asked to write about traumatic experiences reported more positive moods and

---

17 Frederiksen, Yoon, "The effect of expressive writing intervention for infertile couples: a randomized controlled trial" *Human Reproduction*, Volume 32, Issue 2, 1 February 2017, pp. 391–402.

fewer illnesses than students who were assigned to write about superficial experiences.[18]

I recommend trying to write every day—or at least a few times per week—without forcing yourself to write for a certain number of minutes. Either a paper and pen or computer is fine. Start by letting the thoughts flow in a stream-of-consciousness style or have a theme, like, "Things I'm Grateful For." Your ovaries may have refused to be hijacked by stimulation medications and produce a dozen eggs, but expressing gratitude that you have ovaries that are trying to do their best is a positive emotion worth documenting. Write freely, without censoring or critiquing your work. In the words of the poet William Wordsworth, "Fill your paper with the breathings of your heart."

There can be some contraindications to journaling. If it results in self-absorption and becomes a vehicle for going over the same negative thoughts rather than seeing solutions, it may be counterproductive. An option is to try journaling with prompts that give you a specific topic like, "What scares me?" "Who are the people I most admire?" or "What are my short-term goals?" Beth, a second-grade teacher who had suffered many setbacks during her IVFs, turned to journaling but felt that "rehashing my day or just spilling out all my thoughts was anxiety-producing and left me unsettled. It wasn't until I found a journal with prompts that I found journaling enjoyable and mentally helpful. I learned what I value and where I want to go in this one crazy life we have."

New York Times writer Haley Phelan was in an unhappy relationship and her career was stalled when she started to journal.

---

18 Pennebaker, James, *Opening UP: The Healing Power of Expressing Emotion*, Third edition. 2016

Over the next two years her "life completely changed" and she "began a new, fulfilling relationship, enrolled in an MFA Program, and rekindled my freelance writing career." She said she can't know exactly how journaling helped her but said, "Certainly, I got to know the dusty corners of my brain better, and, when I did, my true desires became harder to ignore."

While trying to start your family, you may have pushed important issues into the corners of your mind in order to focus on your goal of having a baby. Looking at your pre-family-building goals and writing about them may help restore you and put you back in touch with the person you were before your loss and frustration.

I like to blog. Does that count as writing?

Sure. There is even some research that shows "Blogging can have a positive impact on psychological consequences experienced by women in fertility treatment."[19]

However, you may choose not to put deeply personal thoughts on a blog, making a private journal a better outlet for them. Patients have told me that they feel sad or angry when someone brags on a blog about falling pregnant "without even trying," so make sure that you don't create leaks in your emotional bucket by spending too much time reading unhelpful blogs.

19 Orr, Elizabeth. "Understanding the Blogging Practices of Women Undergoing In Vitro Fertilization (IVF): A Discourse Analysis of Women's IVF Blogs" *The Qualitative Report*; (Aug 2017): 2206-2230

Green time and forest bathing

THE ANCIENT TAOIST PHILOSOPHERS BELIEVED THAT, as human beings, we are just another part of nature, like the trees, flowers, rivers, oceans, and mountains around us. This intrinsic connection with nature runs through Native American wisdom as well. In Traditional Chinese Medicine theories, the universal energy (Qi) that we all share is enhanced when we breathe in the aromas of the forest or bathe in the ocean. We are sustained and nourished by the time we spend in gardens, fields, forests, and oceans.

While this sounds ethereal and poetic, trading some screen time for green time has proven physical and emotional benefits.

You don't need to commit to walking the Appalachian Trail to commune with nature. Roger S. Ulrich, an environmental psychologist, professor, and founder of the Center for Health Systems Design, found that "simply viewing certain photos of nature can significantly ameliorate stress within five minutes or less . . . Looking at nature scenes rather quickly produces mood improvement and physiological changes such as lower blood pressure and reduced heart rate."[20] His research, and that of other scientists, has shown that patients in hospital rooms with windows and sun coming in heal faster and use less pain medication than patients in windowless rooms. This effect has even been seen when rooms without windows have landscape art on the walls.

Although just looking out a window or at a landscape painting can increase your sense of tranquility and calmness and enhance healing, actually being out in nature is even better. According to the Environmental Protection Agency, Americans spend 93% of their time indoors. My first reaction to this statistic was "No, I am outside much more than that even living through the harsh winters of the Midwest." Then I realized that, on that particular day, I had driven to the gym, back home to change, driven to my office, worked all day, stopped at the store, and then had gone home for the evening. I hadn't spent much time outside at all, and a day like that is common for many people. If you cannot manage to be outside much during the workweek, weekends can work just fine. The Japanese have been promoting a wonderful way to spend weekend time. It is called *shinrinyoku. Shinrin* means "forest," and *yoku* translates to "bathing."

You don't really mean dragging a tub out to a forest preserve, do you?

No, it is not about being in a tub. It means spending time in a forest, soaking up its sounds, smells, air, and textures.

---

20 Ulrich R, "Effects of exposure to nature and abstract pictures on patients recovering from open-heart surgery." *J Soc Psychophysiol Res* 1993; 30:7

The Japanese have meticulously studied and promoted *shinrinyoku* as a way of de-stressing, promoting calmness, and raising one's spirits. A comprehensive study done at the Nippon Medical School showed that participants in forest bathing lowered their blood pressure and adrenalin (high numbers being associated with stress) and improved their immune function, as evidenced by increase in activity of natural killer cells.[21]

Shinrinyoku is about meandering through a forest or park and being mindful of what our senses are experiencing. Our sense of smell may be particularly important while forest bathing. Substances known as phytoncides, organic compounds emitted by pine and cedar trees into forest air, are believed to be responsible for the therapeutic effects of forest bathing. When you are walking and breathing in the air, stop to touch the bark of a tree or the dew on a leaf, or dip your fingers in a stream.

Walking in a prairie or field might not expose you to cedar trees but could have the same positive effects as a forest because it would provide the opportunity to be less shaded by trees and experience more sunlight. Sunlight activates our vitamin D and may increase brain chemicals involved in mood and sleep. Florence Nightingale observed in her *Notes on Nursing* more than 160 years ago, "It is the unqualified result of all of my experience with the sick, that second only to their need of fresh air is their need of light . . . and it is not only light but direct sun-light that they want. People think that the effect is upon the spirits only. This is by no means the case. The sun is not only a painter but a sculptor."

---

21 Li, Qing "Effect of forest bathing trips on human immune function," *Environmental Health and Preventive Medicine*. 2010 Jan; 15(1):9-17

Although it seems easy to be with trees, if you feel that you want some guidance or coaching, there are actually "forest therapy guides" available, mostly on the West and East coasts. You can check with the Association of Nature and Forest Therapy (https://www.natureandforesttherapy.earth) about guides in your area. However, I think you will do just fine walking on your own. I included the information on guides to show you that forest therapy is really a thing.

If your work schedule and family life make it a challenge to find a forest or field to walk in on a daily basis, consider taking a traditional bath at the end of your day, the benefits of which include muscle relaxation, improved circulation, lower blood pressure, and falling asleep faster.

I am so tired of trying things. I just want a magic bullet for feeling better. Any passive tools?

The insertion of small, fine needles, as in acupuncture, is about as passive a therapy as you can get.

There are many studies on the positive effects of acupuncture on mood and the stress relief that acupuncture provides. Dr. Charles Engel, of Walter Reed Army Hospital, studied Post Traumatic Stress Disorder in returning Gulf War vets and found significant positive benefits when acupuncture was added to their treatment plans.[22] Veterans were assigned to receive either anti-anxiety and anti-depression medications, or psychotherapy, both of which are considered usual but only "modestly effective" care. A third group received one of the two traditional treatments (either meds

22 Engel, C, Randomized effectiveness trial of a brief course of acupuncture for posttraumatic stress disorder, Med Care, 2014 Dec;52(12 Suppl 5):S57-64.

or therapy) with the addition of auricular (ear) acupuncture. (It would have been unethical to withhold a proven treatment to people suffering from PTSD, which is why the acupuncture was added to the standard treatments as opposed to acupuncture being researched as a stand-alone treatment.) "Compared with usual care, acupuncture was associated with significantly greater decreases in PTSD symptoms . . . and these improvements were maintained through the 12-week follow-up," according to the study's author, Dr. Charles Engel. "Symptoms of pain and depression also significantly improved in the acupuncture group compared to the usual-care group."[23] This and similar research have resulted in the military making acupuncture available to veterans in their care facilities.

Having a negative pregnancy test month after month or losing a pregnancy after the joy of a positive test can result in some of the same symptoms of PTSD—depression, anxiety, and insomnia. In fact, one study showed that receiving a diagnosis of infertility was rated as stressful as receiving a diagnosis of cancer.[24] I believe that many of my patients suffer from *Present* Traumatic Stress Disorder as they try to do their job, be a good spouse, and pay the bills at the same time they are starting another round of fertility medication and traveling to multiple ultrasound appointments.

Are you saying getting my ears poked with needles can help me feel calmer and stop stressing?

Yes. In short, because the points where needles are placed possibly tap into the nervous system. What follows is the long explanation

---

23 *Ibid.*

24 "The Psychological impact of infertility and its treatment," *Harvard Health Letter*, May 2009

of how this all works, so feel free to skip it if you are not interested in the Western and Eastern view of how acupuncture works.

Acupuncture works because of its effects on the nervous system, which is made up of the brain, spinal cord, sympathetic, parasympathetic, and peripheral nerves. As I mentioned earlier, when the sympathetic system is stimulated, heart rate, blood pressure, and respirations increase, muscles tense, and the adrenal glands start to pump out cortisol. When the parasympathic system is in charge, heart rate, blood pressure, and respirations decrease, muscles relax, and cortisol production decreases. The outer ear has many tiny parasympathetic nerves making it possible that the insertion of needles there stimulates this relaxation response. As I mentioned earlier, there is good evidence that Mindful Meditation also stimulates the parasympathetic system and ratchets down the sympathetic system.

I've read that there are hundreds of specific points. How did the ancients figure out where all of those points are and what problems they help?

First of all, they had a few thousand years to figure it out. I am more intrigued by the fact that people figured out a way for me to ask my phone where the nearest Mexican restaurant is, and that was accomplished in only the last several years. I can imagine that trial, error, and observation over a few thousand years was key.

If you want to receive acupuncture care, it is important to find a skilled practitioner. Like nurses, doctors, plumbers, or teachers, not all acupuncturists are created equal. There are great ones, good ones, mediocre ones, and bad ones. The basic requirement to legally practice acupuncture is state licensure, usually abbreviated

"L.Ac.," short for "Licensed in Acupuncture." Licensure requires graduation from an accredited acupuncture school and passing a national exam. Certification in acupuncture is voluntary and requires continuing-education credits. While licensure is required for practice, do not choose a practitioner solely based on additional credentials or a slick website. The very best way to find a good acupuncturist is to get a personal recommendation by asking your friends and family if they have been *successfully* treated by an acupuncturist they liked.

Getting acupuncture sounds great, but it would be one more thing to fit into my schedule. And it's not covered by insurance, right? It is not universally covered, although some insurance companies have negotiated lower fees for their customers with a restricted list of acupuncturists. I have never had a problem with payment when patients use flex spending or health-savings-account money.

I agree—you don't need one more thing on your schedule. But when you are trying to regain calm, you must make yourself a priority. You accomplish this by setting aside house and community work and leaving work early or arriving later on some days, which, sadly, teachers and shift workers cannot easily do.

It's okay to combine some strategies to make the most of your time. Sit outside near a tree to get your green time and meditate, write, draw, paint, knit, or create something. Power down your digital devices, and read a paperback book instead of skimming your newsfeeds. Listen to a song from start to finish instead of hitting "next" halfway through. This return to analog may not add time to the clock, but it will make time seem to pass more slowly and reduce low-grade anxiety. Cal Newport, Professor of

Computer Science at Georgetown University, presents a compelling argument for the emotional benefits of powering down in his book *Digital Minimalism*. He recommends removing apps like Instagram, Facebook, and Twitter and spending less time with things that "invade your cognitive landscape." At the very least, don't be afraid to turn off notifications or simply call a friend.

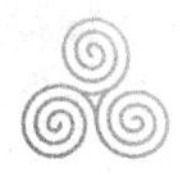

Renourishing Your Body

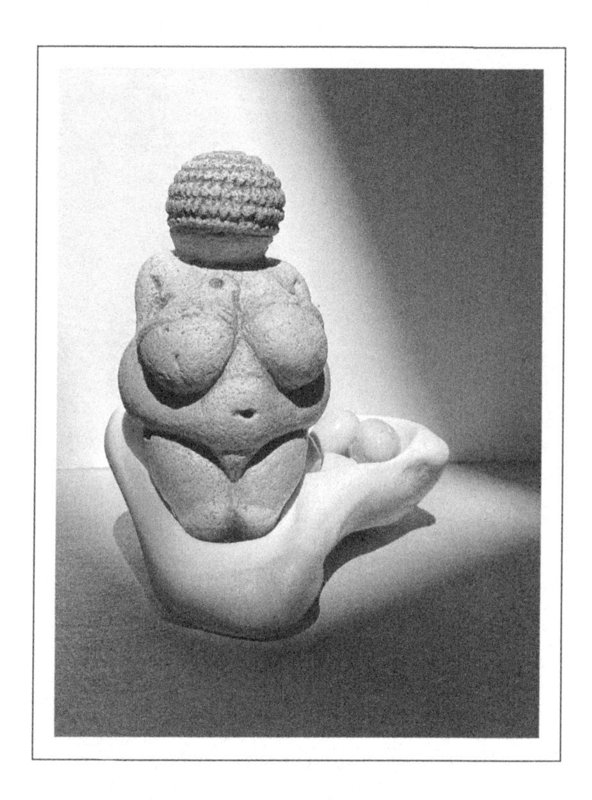

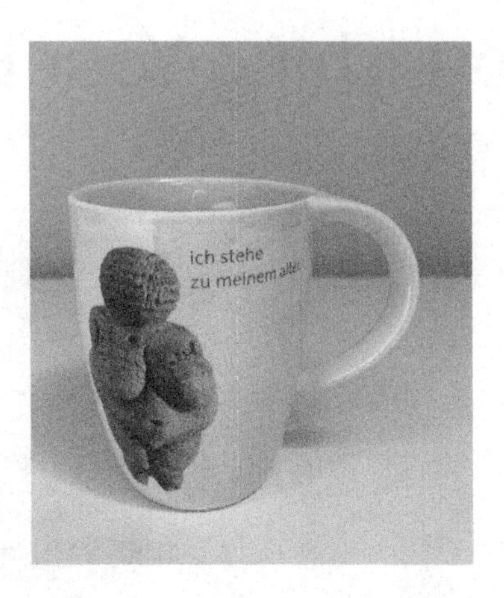

The goddess sculpture on the previous page and on the cup above was found in Austria. Called the Venus of Willendorf, she is believed to be 25,000-year-old and is only 4.3 inches tall. She looks similar to in size and shape of dozens of other fertility sculptures that have been unearthed from all seven continents. These corpulent statues were meant to symbolize the importance of being well nourished for good fertility.

A conversation over tea

I paired Green Tea with this section because substances in green tea renew the body by scooping up cell waste products known as oxidants, earning it the title "anti-oxidant." Only leaves from the camellia sinensis plant can technically be called tea. The way it is harvested, roasted, and fermented determines whether it is called green, black, white or oolong. All these varieties have potential health benefits. Although there are not enough carefully controlled studies to conclusively prove beliefs that green tea is anti-inflammatory, neuroprotective, anti-microbial, cancer reducing and cardiovascular enhancing, the fact remains that the body needs anti-oxident activity for good health. A Rishi Tea Company blurb sums it up best: "The benefits of tea are realized when consumed as part of a healthy lifestyle, on a regular basis, over periods of time."

Does green tea extract in a smoothie have the same benefits?
Sorry but no. There is some evidence that consuming concentrated forms or "extracts" of green tea can cause liver damage. Best to avoid "concentrated" anything, unless it is a researched, prescribed medication. Try a good, organic brand of green tea, and read about steeping methods, as that can influence flavor and bitterness.

A conversation over tea

All healing starts with the mouth

ACUPUNCTURE, STRESS REDUCTION, and nutrition counseling are the main pillars of my approach to self-care. Of these, I believe nutrition, or *nourishment*, as I like to refer to it, is the most important. Dr. Andrew Weil likes to say, that "All healing starts with the mind." I like to say, "All healing starts with the mouth."

"The patient who neglects his diet wastes his doctor's time" is an ancient Chinese proverb. Witch doctor Jane Gleeson's proverb is, "Eat what makes you feel happy—just not too much of it. And be sure to include seven or more servings of fruits and vegetables a day, whether they make you happy or not."

I know you know how to eat well. But you may lose your motivation to eat well if you have been making good food choices all along and you still don't have your baby. What follows is a review and update of best practices in Western and Eastern nutrition, as well as questions that you have frequently asked.

I truly believe Mother Nature, in her excellent planning, put all the plants and animals on this Earth that we need to be healthy and to heal. We just need to find them and eat them. The *food-as-medicine* movement is not new, as plants have sustained us as a species for millennia.

Nutrition is so important for healing and health that I require all patients to send me a one-week food log so I can essentially peer into their cupboards as the ancient Chinese doctors did. Although logs for just a week are a snapshot in time, we tend to eat the same foods and amounts week after week. After years of looking at hundreds of food logs, I have learned that what patients put in their mouths, or, more often, what they *do not* put in their mouths, is a big part of the root cause for many health problems.

Topics in this section apply to the general health and fertility of men and women. Research clearly supports that what a man eats and drinks can have a significant effect on his fertility and the health of his offspring.[25] That makes total sense because half of the genes in an embryo come from sperm and half from the egg. I often wish that, when my patients are picking sperm donors, they could look at their food logs as well as their level of education. What fathers eat matters.

It is likely that there have been times when you gained weight, lost weight, tried to eat impeccably, or just said, "The hell with it." But in an effort to keep your healing and rejuvenating on track here, I want to tweak your body of knowledge on nutrition.

---

25 Nassan, Feiby. "Diet and men's fertility: Does diet affect sperm quality?" *Fertility and Sterility*, 2018 Sep;110(4):570-577.

Before we move on to your questions (which are always really good), I want to share some information on what your family-building journey may have taken out of you nutritionally.

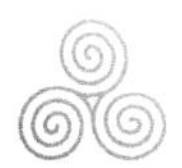

Who stole your nutrients?

SOIL DEPLETION DUE TO FAILURE TO ROTATE CROPS and let dirt rest, along with the breeding of produce for size, growth rate, and pest resistance has resulted in a decrease of nutrients in the fruits and vegetables we eat. U.S. Department of Agriculture data from 1950 to 1999 found "reliable decline" of protein, calcium, phosphorus, iron, and vitamins B2 and C.[26] Although not measured at that time, this is probably the case also for magnesium, zinc, and vitamin B6. This is why I strongly encourage my patients to eat more than the recommended five-to-seven servings of fruits and vegetables today, and to eat organic when they can, because organics tend to be higher in some nutrients.

Even with good nutrition habits, you may have depleted your store of vitamins, minerals, and blood in your efforts to plan a

26 "Dirt Poor: Have Fruits and Vegetables Become Less Nutritious?" *Scientific American*, April 27, 2011

family. Even before you started your journey, environmental and lifestyle factors may have resulted in suboptimal nutrition.

While waiting for the right time to start a family, or for therapeutic purposes, you may have taken oral contraceptives for years. Research indicates that birth control pills "have been shown to affect a number of metabolic and nutritional processes, some insignificantly and others beneficially. The use of contraceptive pills has been shown to decrease the physiologic levels of six nutrients—riboflavin, pyridoxine, folacin, vitamin B12, ascorbic acid, and zinc . . ."[27]

Calcium absorption by bones of adolescent girls can also be impacted by the estrogen in birth-control pills, as indicated by a study published in the *Journal of Endocrinology.* The good news is that the metabolism of vitamin C, iron, copper, and vitamin A may be increased in women who take oral contraceptives.

In addition to the depletion of some vitamins from taking birth-control pills, reproductive years can make you vulnerable to "blood deficiency." This is a Traditional Chinese Medicine (TCM) diagnosis that is sometimes made if a person has a pale tongue, cold hands and feet, trouble sleeping, and heart palpitations. Chronic heavy periods, miscarriages, and blood loss at birth can contribute to "blood deficiency." I want to emphasize that, in TCM, we make a bigger issue of blood loss related to reproductive functions, while modern medicine is not concerned with blood loss unless certain lab values indicate anemia. When I see a patient with a snowy-white tongue who admits to wearing three pairs of socks to bed (or warming her feet on her partner's

---

27 Tyrer, LB, "Nutrition and the Pill," *J Reprod Med.* 1984 Jul;29(7 Suppl):547-50.

back), I suggest she make sure that she has had a complete blood-count check recently.

I had to get tubes and tubes of blood taken while going through fertility treatment. Can that have harmed me?
I often wonder about that, too. Research shows that intensive care unit patients often become anemic (iatrogenic anemia) after a few days, due to multiple blood draws in one day. But you are not likely to have had multiple blood draws on each of several consecutive days, as inpatients often do.

A healthy person has 1,000 mg of iron stores, and your bone marrow is constantly using it to make and store new red blood cells. Anemia will not result until iron stores are depleted.

Whole food is the best way to give your body the building blocks for making blood and avoiding anemia or blood deficiency. You need the iron that is in food. There are two kinds of iron that you need—heme and non-heme—to produce hemoglobin, the oxygen-transporting protein in blood. Meat and some types of fish have mostly heme iron, with a small amount of non-heme. Vegetables, nuts, seeds, and iron-fortified foods have mostly non-heme iron and a small amount of heme. A person needs to eat a large amount of green vegetables to get the amount of heme iron that would be in one small portion of grass-fed beef. I sometimes recommend eating some red meat to get "caught up" to my patients who show consistent signs of blood deficiency and to those vegetarians who are not getting enough plant-based food to nourish iron stores.

When patients have had a history of trouble building up a thick enough lining for an embryo transfer, I share my TCM theory that they might be blood deficient. Women usually get adequate doses of the hormones responsible for building a lining, so it begs the question of why a lining would not grow. My unproven theory is that it could involve the fact that the hormones are traffic directors, not components of blood. They need traffic, that is, blood, to direct. It could be coincidence, but many of the patients I have seen who feared a repeat of a transfer cancellation due to thin lining *did* grow a nice, thick lining before a subsequent transfer after focusing on eating more blood-building and iron-rich foods.

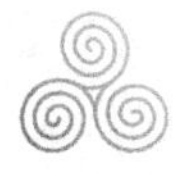

You need to eat only three things

THE THREE MAIN CATEGORIES OF WHOLE FOODS are protein, carbohydrate, and fat. These broad categories are referred to as macronutrients. You need all three to survive and high-quality ones to thrive. They each contain specific vitamins and minerals referred to as micronutrients, because, although they are vital, we need only small amounts of them. Eating a variety of high-quality macros will guarantee that you get the micros. That is all you need to do for Renourishment and future health.

Most whole foods, meaning fruits, vegetables, meat, dairy, and whole grains, contain a combination of protein, carb, and fat, although one category usually predominates. For example, dairy products contain mostly protein and fat, with a smaller amount of carb, and whole grains contain mostly protein and carb, with smaller amounts of fat (think wheat-germ oil). Mother Nature must have known there would come a time when people would try different diets that eliminate one of the food groups, resulting in fat-free and carbohydrate-free diets. So she tucked all three macros into many foods.

A simple way to get all the nutrients you need is to look down at your plate at each meal and ask yourself, *Where is my protein, where is my high-quality carb, and where is my high-quality, healthy fat?* Once you have done that, enjoy your glass of wine with your dinner or your small portion of dessert afterward. Sometimes women apologize for their husbands' eating habits by saying, "He's a meat-and-potatoes guy." A palm-sized portion of lean grass-fed beef with a side of sweet potatoes or white potatoes (not drenched in sour cream) is actually an okay meal. Add a nice, green organic vegetable, and there is no need to apologize.

Although I believe in food-as-medicine and that nutrients are best absorbed from whole foods, there is one nutrient that you should take in pill form to cover all of your bases, especially if you are continuing to try to conceive—and even if you eat a very good diet. Since you have been on a family-building journey for a while, you know I'm talking about vitamin B9, more commonly known as folate. Solid research indicates that a deficiency in folate or its synthetic form, folic acid, may increase the incidence of brain and spinal-cord problems in a developing embryo. Inadequate levels of folate and folic acid have also been associated with—but not proven—miscarriage and infertility.

That has always confused me—am I supposed to take folate or folic acid?

Many of my patients ask that question, because the terms are often used interchangeably.

Folate and folic acid are two forms of the micronutrient vitamin B9, which helps the body use protein and carbohydrate in addition to its role in the formation of DNA and red blood cells. Can't get more important than that. Folate is the natural form of B9, meaning it is found in found in asparagus, deep-green leafy vegetables, beets, citrus fruits, spinach, Brussel sprouts, avocados, bananas, eggs, peas, beans, and chickpeas. Folic acid, the other form of B9, can be synthesized in a laboratory and put into vitamin pills or added to food products like bread and cereal. When you eat foods naturally high in folate or take a folic-acid pill, your body must convert the two forms of B9 (both folate and folic acid) into the only form of B9 that can actually get into cells, called methylfolate.

My sisters both were told that they have a gene problem that causes them to be low in folate. So, I decided to take extra folate, too, since we obviously share genes. Is that okay?
The gene mutation you may be referring to is the one that results in a lack of the enzyme needed to convert B9 (either the folic acid or folate form) into methylfolate, the only form of B9 that can enter cells. The lack of this conversion enzyme, methylenetetrahydrofolate reductase (abbreviated MTHFR) can put a woman at risk for low methyl folate. This, in turn, can put a developing baby at risk for brain and spinal-cord problems and may be a factor in recurrent miscarriage. The science on MTHFR gene mutation and its effects is still evolving, and, in part, the level of concern depends on the gene variant. It's complicated, and, if you have the gene mutation, ask your doctor which form and what amount of B9 you should be taking. A big part of the solution involves being sure to get high-folate foods and taking the recommended amounts of folate and folic-acid supplementation.

Getting back to your question, I don't think you should take extra B9 just because your sister has been diagnosed. You share some, but not all, of her genes. Also, if your body is not absorbing and using the extra folic acid you are taking, it could theoretically build up in the bloodstream and cause problems, so get your doctor's input on this evolving and complicated situation.

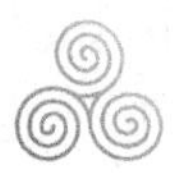

Pop quiz

BEFORE I COACH PATIENTS ON NUTRITION, I like to get a baseline on their food intake. I ask both partners to keep a food log for one week. Even in two-mom couples, where genetic material will be from only one of the women, I want to know the food habits of the family unit. Good nutrition is key to a happy and healthy life, so even if you are not trying to conceive, please try this food-log exercise. If you are trying to conceive, know that an impressive amount of scientific information exists on the effect of a father's lifestyle habits on offspring.[28]

Record everything you eat and drink, with the approximate amounts, for one week. I guarantee that you will get some insight. Most people get enough of the macronutrients protein, carbohydrate, and fat but may not be getting enough micronutrients due to low intake of fruits and vegetables. Western nutrition

28 Finlayson, Judith, *You Are What Your Grandparents Ate: What You Need to Know About Nutrition, Experience, Epigenetics, and the Origins of Chronic Disease*, 2009

recommendations are that we eat a combined total of five to seven servings of fruits and vegetables each day. Some nutritionists advise increasing that number to seven to nine servings per day, because of the decreasing amount of vitamins in fruits and vegetables that I mentioned earlier. Seven servings per day is a good goal. A serving is a half of a cup to a cup, or a whole banana or apple. Current research shows that U.S. daily intake is about one serving of fruit and one-half serving of vegetable. It is not uncommon to go through a new patient' food log and see just two total servings for the week, and they are usually both fruit. It's easy to go through the day and not get the servings you need even if you are eating well. Many people have a fine breakfast of eggs and whole-wheat toast, or oatmeal with milk, and then a turkey-and-cheese sandwich on whole-grain bread for lunch. This is then followed by a piece of fruit and nuts for an afternoon snack, and salmon and broccoli for dinner. Not a bad intake at all, but that is still only one fruit and one vegetable for the day. A deficit of three servings per day becomes 21 servings per week and 84 servings per month.

Some patients who don't eat enough vegetables or fruits have told me they feel confident that they get their vitamins and minerals because they take a daily vitamin pill. The problem is that vitamins in supplements are manufactured synthetically, and some scientists question how much of these synthetic vitamins are absorbed and used by the body. Mother Nature, in her infinite wisdom, designed vitamins and minerals to work together in whole foods, rather than be consumed as separate elements. For example, vitamins A, D, E, and K are present in fat and need fat to be absorbed. If we could get everything we need from a pill, I personally would never grocery shop or cook, neither of which I enjoy. I would just take vitamin pills and eat chocolate chip cookies. I think I would feel awful in a short amount of time.

When my patients increase their fruit and vegetable intake to at least five or six servings per day, they frequently notice in just a few weeks that their hair looks shinier, their skin looks more vibrant, with fewer blemishes, and they feel more energetic. I like to think that the organs we can't see, like kidneys, lungs, and ovaries, are functioning better, too. Although I have always attributed the improvement I see in skin and hair to their increased intake of fruits and vegetables, I read an article recently that meditation also results in skin improvement, possibly due to its cortisol-lowering effects. It doesn't matter whether it is vegetables or meditation—people are always happy to have fewer blemishes.

After recording your intake for a week, see if your combined fruit and vegetable intake is 35 or more. Most of my patients are 30% to 50% low, averaging about two to three servings per day. If you did make quota, congratulations, and keep up the good work.

If you find that after a week you are averaging two servings per day or fewer, it can seem challenging to increase by three to four servings per day. I have some simple guidelines that make it very easy to make quota:

1. Never let a meal go by without a fruit or vegetable. There is nothing wrong with almond milk or yogurt or oatmeal or an egg and toast for breakfast, but enjoy a fruit or vegetable with it. Now you are up to three, assuming you eat three meals a day.

2. Make your mid-morning or mid-afternoon snack a fruit or vegetable. Now you are up to four.

3. Two servings of vegetable (preferably one of them being green) with dinner. Now you are up to five.

4. Take inventory at about three or four each afternoon, and if you have four servings to go to make quota, have some chopped vegetables with your dip at happy hour, or slice an apple to snack on while preparing dinner. If you grab a few chips after that, it's fine.

Try to diversify your choices to ensure you get the full range of vitamins and minerals. The easiest way to do this is to choose a variety of colors—green, deep-green, orange, red, yellow, or purple. If red grapes and asparagus were on sale and you bought a lot, fine—eat them all week, but then switch to cantaloupe or beets the next week.

Should I be eating only organic fruits and vegetables? They do cost more. Will it really make a difference for healing and hormonal balance?

There is a growing body of evidence that avoiding environmental chemicals like pesticides leads to better reproductive and general health for men and women. A 2018 study[29] published in the *Journal of the American Medical Association* clearly showed a significantly

29 Chiu, Y, "Association Between Pesticide Residue Intake from Consumption of Fruits and Vegetables and Pregnancy Outcomes Among Women Undergoing Infertility Treatment with Assisted Reproductive Technology"; *JAMA Intern Med.* 2018;178(1):17-26

higher pregnancy rate and lower miscarriage rate in the women who ate mostly organic fruits and vegetables as opposed to women who ate more servings of non-organic.

Given that reproductive and thyroid hormones are very likely disrupted by toxic chemicals on foods, organic foods offer a good way to decrease your exposure and enhance hormonal balance. But you don't need to blame yourself if you have not always been eating organic as you tried to start your family. Beautiful and smart babies are born every day whose mothers did not eat organic during their pregnancies. The other good news is that prices for organic versus non-organic produce are coming down, as higher demand has led to more availability and more competition. I know you want to do everything you can that might help general health or future fertility, so I strongly encourage you to eat organic produce when you can, especially those favorite fruits and vegetables you eat frequently.

I juice my fruits and veggies—that's OK, right?

Yes and no. Fruit and vegetable juices are good because a lot of nutrients are condensed into a few ounces. But fruit juices can then be high in natural sugar, which is not a big problem unless you are diabetic or trying to keep your calorie count low. The juicing process also removes the fiber from fruits and vegetables, which contain nutrients and slows down the metabolism of sugar in your body.

Try to eat whole fruits and vegetables when you can, and fill in around the sides with juices. Eating more fiber-rich whole fruits and vegetables has helped some of my patients who experienced constipation associated with progesterone supplementation during fertility treatment.

I like fruits and vegetables. What if I ate a totally plant-based diet?
Then you would be called a vegan and probably get a lot of grief from your mother-in-law. Just kidding. If you are married, your mother-in-law is probably wonderful.

When done correctly, following a strict vegan diet (no animal products) has not been associated with reproductive problems. Unfortunately, I often see way too many crackers and cereal bars listed in my vegan patients' food logs and not enough protein, iron-rich foods, and high-quality fats.

There is some research to show that intake of plant protein is associated with better ovulatory function than animal protein.[30] This could be because many plants contain building blocks for hormones called phytoestrogens. If having regular menstrual cycles will help you feel that you are on the road to recovery, regardless of whether you are trying to conceive, eating more plant protein and less animal protein may help you with that goal. Nuts are a great and convenient source of protein and have been shown to decrease the risk of premature death by about 11%. Raw or roasted nuts, as opposed to those saturated in oil and salt, are a better choice.

I think I want to try being a vegan. I remember reading something about needing to eat a certain combination of foods to get "complete proteins." What is the deal with that again?
We get the protein we need from two sources—plants and animals. We need protein for the production of enzymes, blood, hormones, muscles, cartilage, skin, and for proper functioning of the immune system.

30 Willet, Chavarro, and Skerrett, *The Fertility Diet*, 2007, page 93

The amino acids in plants and animal products are the building blocks for protein. There are 20 amino acids; 11 are made by the body, and 9 are "essential," meaning we cannot make them and must get them through food. Meat, fish, eggs and dairy contain these 9 amino-acid building blocks and are therefore called "complete proteins." But most plants, with the exception of whole soy, do not contain all of the amino acids and are, therefore, called "incomplete proteins." You have probably heard that vegetarians need to eat rice and beans to have a complete protein. That is because beans contain none of the essential amino acid methionine, while rice does, and rice contains limited amounts of the essential amino acid lysine but has methionine.

Okay—can you run that by me again?

Eggs, fish, meat, dairy products, and whole soy will provide protein with all the amino acids that are essential. If you are vegan or vegetarian and rely on vegetables, beans, peas, whole grains, nuts, and seeds for your protein, you must eat adequate amounts, in the right combination, to get all the amino acids needed for a healthy protein intake.

How much protein am I supposed to be eating?

In general, women need about 46 grams of protein per day, and men need about 56, although this can differ with age, health status, activity level, and weight. A gram is a measurement of weight, and a chicken breast has 43 grams of protein, an egg has 6, a quarter-pound beef patty has 20, and 6 ounces of Greek yogurt has 12 to 18. If your day included eggs, a serving of fish or meat, milk, nuts, yogurt, cheese, and some whole-grain bread, you have likely covered your protein needs. Eggs or oatmeal for breakfast, a peanut-butter sandwich on whole-grain bread at lunchtime, and a serving (which is about the size of the palm of your hand) of beef, chicken, or fish for dinner would easily provide what you need if you are in the 140-pound range. If you are bigger, pregnant, breast feeding, body building, or recovering from a serious illness, you may need more protein servings.

If you have concerns that you are not getting enough protein, keep track of your intake for a few days. Nutrition-oriented websites list protein content of foods and the amounts you need for your size and age. If you are deficient, I would recommend increasing your intake of protein-rich whole foods before supplementing with protein powder, which will not have as much fiber and vitamins as whole food.

Did you just tell me a few paragraphs ago that soy is in the fish, meat, egg, and dairy category of complete proteins?
Yes, I did.

Don't some people say that soy is bad for women?
Yes, they do.

Soy has gotten a bad rap because it contains "phytoestrogens," or plant-based, estrogen-like compounds, and there is concern about their effect on a woman's hormonal function. Medical researchers have concluded that soy can have either estrogenic or anti-estrogenic effects on the body, depending on ethnicity, menopause status, and whether the soy is fermented or unfermented. Fermentation is a process in which soybeans are aged with microorganisms and bacteria that break down some of the compounds of concern. Fermented soy is used to make miso, tempeh, and most types of tofu. Unfermented soy is used in soy cheese, soy burgers, soy milk, soy baby formula, and many other processed food products. It is these unfermented sources of soy that may be affecting a person's hormones. As with all foods, the amount consumed probably determines what effects a person might experience, so if you want to enjoy a soy latte, go ahead. Just don't have soy milk on your breakfast cereal, soy latte for morning break, soy yogurt for lunch, soy protein bar for an afternoon snack, and soy cheese at Happy Hour. I have seen five servings of soy a day and for most days of the week in a patient's food log.

I like edamame. That's just another name for soybeans, right?
Soybeans are the mature beans, and edamame are the young, green, unripe beans. Interestingly, soybeans contain much more protein and other nutrients than the young edamame.

Bottom line: soy is a great source of protein, unsaturated fats, B vitamins, potassium, and magnesium. Just eat fermented soy when you can and limit your intake of unfermented soy.

I don't like soy or meat very much, so I put protein powder in my smoothie and usually have a protein bar for lunch. That's okay—right?
It would be better to get your protein from whole food. Powders and bars are often flavored with sugars (adding calories) and when the powder is derived from animal hooves it can have a high rate of heavy-metal contamination, according to the Clean

Labels Project. You can find good information at the website www.cleanlabelproject.org.

My patient Ellen had no trouble conceiving but had suffered three miscarriages. She was understandably ambivalent about conceiving again, and felt that adding collagen powder to her oatmeal and smoothies might boost her health. Although there is some research indicating that collagen might improve hair and fingernails, many nutritional scientists agree that we know little about its absorption and benefits for other parts of the body. A look at Ellen's food log for a week clearly showed that, between her intake of eggs (seven in a week), oatmeal, yogurt, sprouted grains, walnuts, cottage cheese, chicken (two servings in a week), and some shredded beef in Mexican food, she ate plenty of protein. Her intake of protein from animal sources was well balanced by her good intake of plant-based protein from sweet potatoes, beans, peanut butter, and kale. She was consuming about five servings of vegetables and fruits per day, and although six or seven would be better, she was getting small amounts of protein in these servings. Ellen did not need to add collagen protein powder to her smoothies and oatmeal. Look at your protein intake before reaching for supplements, and choose organic, whole-food sources when you can. Increase plant-based whole foods like soybeans and its fermented products tofu and tempeh, chickpeas (think hummus), lentils, hempseed, green peas, peanuts, quinoa, hemp seeds, chia seeds, and potatoes. FYI: vegan sources of protein powder are made from peas, soybeans, hemp, pumpkin seeds, chia seeds, and brown rice.[31]

---

31 http://www.health.harvard.edu/staying-healthy/the-hidden-dangers-of-protein-powders

Not all of these are "complete proteins," so blends of the plant sources are recommended if you are consuming powders. Once again, really try to get your protein from whole foods rather than isolated proteins.

If I get enough protein, can I eliminate carbs to lose the weight I put on while trying to get pregnant?
You can lower carbs but not eliminate them.

Your body converts carbohydrates into glucose for the energy your body needs. If you do not have any carbs on board, your body will break down fat for fuel, which may lead to weight loss. But there is a downside. The fat will break down into ketones, and high levels of ketones over long periods of time can harm organs as well as cause fatigue, nausea, and headaches. In addition to this, if you eliminate carbs, you will be missing key nutrients in some whole grains and carbohydrate-containing fruits and vegetables. It is not surprising that research shows that extreme no-carb diets are difficult to stick to, because fruits and starchy vegetables are limited, and no grains, beer, wine, or pasta are allowed on these diets. Initial weight loss can be impressive, but research shows that long-term weight loss is no better than with other types of diets.

If you want to cut carbs, start by reducing the bad ones found in pastries, donuts, candy, pretzels, white bread, and other processed food items. These are low-quality sources of carb because they are calorie dense and made with flour and sugar that have been stripped of their nutrients in processing. Enjoy high-quality, nutrient-dense whole-food carbs like quinoa, oats, brown rice, oats, buckwheat, and sweet potatoes. Whole-grain breads are a good source, but most commercial products are a mixture of white and whole-grain flour. Bananas, mangoes, and apples, are considered high-carb fruits but contain so many great vitamins that you should keep them in your diet even when looking for low-carb fruits. Just eat them in moderation, and stock up on the lower-carb fruits like blueberries, raspberries, peaches, honeydew melon, and cantaloupe. Be mindful of dried fruits, as their carb content (in the form of natural sugar) does not shrink with their size.

Enjoy quality carbs. Mother Nature wants you to and has provided many to choose from.[32]

So, I can enjoy pasta again?
Yes! Pasta made from durum wheat or whole grain is high in protein, low in fat, is digested slowly, and is usually fortified with folic acid, making it part of healthy eating. As with potatoes, it is the toppings of cheese, meat, and cream sauces that can pack on the calories. Extra virgin olive oil, tomato sauces, sautéed vegetables, and a little salt and pepper is the best way to enjoy your pasta. If you have not tried soba noodles, which are made from buckwheat (which is naturally gluten free), go for it.

Okay, so I can cut out fat instead of carbohydrate to lose weight?
No. You can reduce it if you are eating too much, but fat is your friend, not your foe. What follows is my big fat advice about fat.

Of the three macronutrients required for life, fat is my personal favorite. When we eat fat and sugar, Mother Nature designed our

---

32 https://www.mayoclinic.org/healthy-lifestyle/weight-loss/in-depth/low-carb-diet/art-20045831

brain circuits to light up and signal "reward," something similar to what happens with opiate ingestion.[33]

This could have been Mother Nature's way of ensuring that we get an adequate intake of fat, since it is needed for important cell and organ function.

Fat is a major component of cell membranes, nerve sheaths, and hormones. Cholesterol, a type of fat, is a major component of estrogen and progesterone. Women athletes and anorexic women often stop menstruating because they lack the dietary and body fat necessary for hormone production. If your goal is to have or return to normal periods, fat is an important nutrient. If you are planning to conceive, your developing baby will need fat to make all cell membranes and the protective covering for brain cells. Regardless of whether you will be trying to conceive, you need fat to absorb the vitamins A, D, E, and K, the so-called "fat-soluble vitamins."

In an effort to counteract the weight gain from hormone supplementation or pregnancy, my patients often cut their fat intake too much.

This was the case with Kristen, a patient whose physician advised her to lose weight to increase her chances of a successful embryo transfer. She committed to losing weight and ate little to no fat. When I explained that eating a balanced diet at this important time included healthy fats, she replied, "Have you seen this hip? There is plenty of fat there!" However, I explained that the embryo baby she would soon have on board wouldn't be able to leave the womb, take a bite out of her hip, and return safely to the "Palace for the Baby," as the ancient Chinese called

---

33 Avena NM, "Evidence for sugar addiction: Behavioral and neurochemical effects of intermittent, excessive sugar intake," *Neurosci Biobehav Rev.*, 2008; 31: 20-39

the uterus. Although she would have plenty of progesterone from her injections for the first trimester, she needed to give her body and placenta the ingredients to take over the job of hormone production in the second trimester, when hormone injections are discontinued.

Although we can assume that the fat needed for the natural production of hormones comes from dietary intake, it is interesting to note that babies *in utero* may be borrowing a bit of fat from a mother's brain as they grow. *The Journal of Neuroradiology* published an interesting study in which women's brains were MRI'd before, during, and after pregnancy. A reduction in brain size was evident six months into pregnancy. Fortunately, by six months post-partum, the brain size was back to pre-pregnancy size. The brain is the fattiest organ in the body, at 60% fat. The cells that shrink during pregnancy and then fluff up again after pregnancy are largely made up of "lipid" tissue, which is a form of fat. Perhaps this cell shrinkage is the body utilizing cell fat to obtain the components needed for hormone production or the proper fats needed for baby's brains. (This possible explanation about why the brain shrinks was total speculation on my part, and you will find no support of it in the literature. I am always trying to think of the Creator's reasons for natural phenomena.)

Please know that I understand your choice to cut even healthy dietary fat to lose weight. This idea has been programmed into us. But research does not support that cutting fat intake, except as part of reducing total calorie intake, makes a difference. "Despite the pervasive dogma that one needs to cut fat from their diet to lose weight, the existing scientific evidence does not support low-fat diets over other dietary interventions for long-term weight loss."[34]

Okay, you have convinced me to eat good fats. Can you give me that Good Fat, Bad Fat list again?

Sure, and I will try to keep it simple, because I know you have read all this before.

Good fats include olive, canola, and safflower oil, avocados, most nuts, most seeds, and most fish, with salmon and olive oil being superstars. Coconut oil is trending right now as a "good" fat, but it contains a combination of saturated ("bad") fat and medium-chain triglycerides, which are probably a "good" fat. The pros and cons of this mixture need more research, so, for now, don't overdo it on coconut oil.

These sources of good fats are referred to as mono- and polyunsaturated fats. They protect the body from heart disease by raising the level of HDL, the "good" cholesterol. Note: when trying to remember the difference between HDL and LDL cholesterol, I tell people, "H' is for *Helper*—and you want it *High*—and "L" is for *Lousy*—and you want it *Low*.

But I should avoid eggs, right? Because the yoke has cholesterol, and that's bad for the heart.

No! Eggs are a near-perfect food with small amounts of almost every nutrient you need. The white part is a great source of protein, and the yoke has iron, vitamins A, B, D, and E, and calcium, zinc, lutein, and selenium.

34 https://www.hsph.harvard.edu/news/press-releases/low-fat-diet-not-most-effective-in-long-term-weight-loss/

Eggs do have some cholesterol in them, but your liver is making cholesterol every day (often out of saturated fat). When you eat cholesterol, your liver will simply make less for the day. Seventy percent of people will not see any change in their lipid (blood-fat) numbers from eating eggs and can eat as many as seven eggs per week without increasing their risk of cardiovascular disease.[35]

Sources of fat to be enjoyed in limited amounts are the saturated fats in meat, whole milk, cream, butter, cheese, coconut products, and palm oil. There are good nutrients in these foods (iron in meat, protein in dairy), so it really is okay to eat them. However, too much saturated fat can raise LDL cholesterol, increasing the risk of cardiovascular disease.

A good guideline is that the intake of saturated fat should not exceed about 10% of your total caloric intake. For a 2000-calorie diet, about 20 grams of saturated fat should be the limit. That is the approximate amount in 8 pats of butter, three glasses of whole milk, or a typical burger and fries. A Burger King Whopper and Fries has about 14 grams of saturated fat, and a McDonald's cheeseburger and fries about 8.5 grams, according to their websites. While it is nice to know that you can enjoy fast food on occasion, it is the total nutrition picture that is important when trying to lose weight, and the meal from Burger King is about 900 calories. McDonald's lists a cheeseburger and fries as about 680 calories.

The really bad fats to be avoided are trans fats. These are plant-based oils that were perfectly good oils until they were tampered with in the food lab by adding a hydrogen atom onto its chain

---

35 https://www.mayoclinic.org/dont-get-tricked-by-these-3-heart-health-myths/art

of molecules. This made the oils solid at room temperature and, therefore, more useful in commercial baked goods. Renamed "partially hydrogenated oils," they both raise bad cholesterol and lower good cholesterol, markedly increasing the risk of cardiovascular disease. There is no reason for you to consume them. European countries started banning them way back in 2004 (Denmark was the first), and most other European countries followed. The U.S. did not ban trans fats until 2018 but extended the deadline to 2020. So, depending on how old the frozen pie crusts and breaded shrimp in your freezer is, you may own food with partially hydrogenated fat in it. Protect yourself by reading food labels before purchasing an item.

If you want to cut a "food" from your diet to lose weight and feel better, zero in on white sugar, a processed form of carbohydrate.

I know I eat too much sugar. How do I break that habit?

I am proud of you for wanting to reduce added processed sugar. You can try going cold turkey, but that's difficult.

We are wired to crave sugar, perhaps for survival, as breast milk tastes very sweet. Functional brain MRI imaging shows that sugar lights up the same reward circuits as narcotics. I admit to being a sugar-holic. I eat vegetables I don't like because I know they are good for me, but I have never met a cookie that I didn't like. Some days I feel like sugar is one of my macronutrients, because it is where most of my calories have come from.

In addition to its non-nutritive calories, too much processed sugar may cause an inflammatory response in the body. It is associated with an increased risk of diabetes, cardiovascular disease, and depression.

I am not overly concerned about your intake of the natural forms of sugar in fresh fruit, unless you are diabetic, in which case, you need to be aware of your total added and natural sugar intake. Try to stay under about 24 grams of sugar per day, which would be about 6 teaspoons (1 teaspoon = 4 grams). Most processed-food labels will list sugar content in grams, but most people can visualize sugar better in teaspoons, which labels don't list. Soft drinks have about 9 teaspoons, fruit juices and energy drinks about 8 teaspoons, and protein and cereal bars about 5 teaspoons. This one got me: one tablespoon of ketchup has one teaspoon of sugar. If you want to have all your teaspoons for the day in one serving of something you enjoy, go ahead, but then adjust. That is, have that piece of cake at the office birthday party, but have a white-wine spritzer instead of a sugary margarita at Happy Hour. And don't be afraid to scrape some of the frosting off the cake. Nobody cares.

As you read labels to determine grams of sugar in a product, it is not a good sign if it is listed as the first or second ingredient. Although we think of white table sugar or cane sugar when we read labels, processed forms include fructose, glucose, malt syrup, corn syrup, high-fructose corn syrup, and others. Another important label-reading tip: ingredients like calories and grams of sugar are often listed as "per serving" to trick us into thinking a product doesn't have much in it. I am no longer shocked when I see three chips listed as a serving.

I'm not suggesting that you *have* to give up sweets, but give some thought to how eating sugar makes you want to eat more. When your insulin rises to digest sugar, it can do its job so well that your blood sugar falls and you are hungry again. Hence the craving for more sugar. Try slowing down the jolt of white sugar to your system by having some milk or an apple with your cookies.

What about artificial sweeteners?

I'm not a big fan of artificial sweeteners, due to the controversial evidence linking them to health problems, so I would rather see you use a little honey here and there rather than the artificial stuff. Even stevia, which comes from a plant, goes through a lot of "processing" that can render it unhealthy.

I know I need to cut down on sugar. Do I have to give up caffeine, too?

That depends on how much you drink and how sensitive you are to it.

Most of us get our caffeine from coffee, although there is caffeine in green tea and chocolate made from cacao beans. The upside of coffee is that the beans are rich in antioxidants, which are needed to move waste products from cells. But the caffeine in the beans is a vasoconstrictor, which results in a higher heart rate and blood pressure, both of which can put one at risk for cardiovascular disease. Jolts of caffeine given to pregnant mice have been shown to constrict tiny blood vessels, including ones feeding the placenta. My advice is to avoid jolting your body by limiting your intake to one to two cups per day. There is 75 to 200 mg of caffeine per cup, depending on the beans and brewing methods. Green tea has about 30 to 40 mg of caffeine per cup. If you feel jittery or notice palpitations after whatever amount you drink, your body may be telling you something. If moderate amounts agree with you, enjoy it, but reduce the risk of a caffeine jolt by not drinking it on an empty stomach. I don't drink coffee after breakfast—if I do, I don't sleep well. I was disappointed to learn that the iced dragon fruit tea from a popular coffee chain that I chugged recently had an added 75mg of caffeine. Who would have guessed?

If you will be continuing to try to conceive, or if you have suffered a miscarriage, do not stress about caffeine in moderation. Although I have had many patients tell me, "I didn't get pregnant until I cut out caffeine," the research does not definitively (there are both positive and negative studies) support a cause-and-effect relationship between fertility and moderate amounts of caffeine.

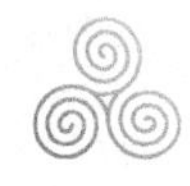

Bad habits and good habits

HAVING LOOKED AT HUNDREDS OF PATIENT FOOD LOGS in the past 25 years, here are the bad eating habits trending right now that are easy to replace with good habits.

Lack of diversity in food choices

This can result in a lack of diversity in nutrients. It's common to see the same fruits and vegetables week after week in patients' food logs. I often hear, "Potatoes are the only vegetable my husband will eat." Many of us tend to shop for and eat the same foods, with bananas, chicken, and oatmeal leading the pack. There's absolutely nothing wrong with those foods, but there is a reason Mother Nature put so many varieties of plants and animals on the planet. Use this time of Renourishment to have fun trying new whole foods. Perhaps every time you grocery shop, set a goal of buying one fruit or vegetable that is new to you or that you don't often eat.

Too many sport drinks

Besides the freakish color of your tongue after drinking one, sport drinks are high in sugar and bottled in plastic, the dangers of which we will talk about later. In 2012, *The British Medical Journal* investigated sport drinks and concluded that, with the possible exception of elite athletes, they do not hydrate the average active person any better than plain water does. It's the same story for "vitamin" and "fitness" waters, where the nutrients in them do not necessarily meet your daily requirements. Even bottled tea may not be healthy—a popular brand lists itself as "Just a Tad Sweet" and has 25 grams of sugar, the equivalent of six teaspoons of sugar.

Too many cereal bars

There is nothing wrong with having one as an afternoon snack, but using them on a daily basis as a substitute for a balanced meal will deprive you of the opportunity for fresh fruits and vegetables. They can also be high in calories and sugar. Some high-protein bars have nearly 400 calories as opposed to a banana at 110, an apple at 130, and an orange at 80 calories. If you enjoy cereal bars, eat one after eating an apple.

Portions of healthy food that are too small

I often see that someone records four grapes or half an apple. Eat the whole apple, or have a cup of grapes and get the advantage of more of the nutrients Mother Nature has put in them.

Portions that are too big

Eating in restaurants is a risk factor here. It is easier to control portions when you cook at home, but when you are presented with a large plate of pasta or meat with fries on the side, it is hard not to eat it, often for fear of wasting it. Don't be hesitant to split an entrée with your dinner partner, or bring half home. You just cut your calories (and bill) by half. If you request a container to bring some of your food home, try not to leave it on the table like I usually do.

Not enough good fat

I have already mentioned the necessity and benefits of healthy fats in your diet, and that reducing fats too much is extremely common among my patients who are trying to lose weight.

Wasting time on fad diets

So many diets out there—Adkins, South Beach, Ketogenic, Paleo, Zone, Cabbage Soup, Baby Food, Raw Food, Lemon Detox, etc., etc. While we all know people who lost weight on some of these diets, research shows that most will gain it back and that severely restricted diets are very difficult to stick to. The easiest way to spot a fad diet that may drain instead of nourish you are claims that seem too good to be true, diets that involve a supplement you must buy, and diets that eliminate one of the three macronutrients protein, carbohydrate, or fat. I call these the "No Diets." No meat, no dairy, no gluten, no alcohol, etc.

If you are allergic to certain foods or you notice that you feel better when you don't eat gluten or dairy, then, of course, don't eat them. Just make sure you get your calcium and high-quality carb from other sources. Other dietary trends like intermittent fasting "have been shown to be no more effective for weight loss than other types of diets and, in fact, may lead to muscle loss."[36] Raw-food diets deprive you of some of the nutrients released from fruits and vegetables during the cooking process, like lycopene and beta-carotene. However, cooking can decrease the amount of vitamins C and B in food, so the best approach is to eat both cooked and uncooked fruits and vegetables.

The good habits that will help you stay well-nourished are:

Make smoothies

You can easily pack in at least three servings of fruits and vegetables in a smoothie. Consider not using all raw ingredients by steaming or sautéing some of the vegetables you use because this makes them easier to digest. Throw in last night's dinner vegetable leftovers. The "stomach qi" or energy, as we call it in ancient Eastern nutrition, can be depleted a bit if it has to always break down fiber to get at nutrients.

Prepare vegetables and fruits in advance

Having vegetables washed and chopped in advance makes it easy to throw them into your scrambled eggs or on top of your store-bought pizza. Although some types of berries don't last as long if you pre-wash them, many will be fine and convenient to grab for yogurt, cereal, and peanut-butter sandwiches. My favorite trick with cilantro is to wash it, dry it, and put it in a glass of water in the refrigerator. It lasts for a week without wilting as an easy add-on for eggs, sandwiches, and baked potatoes.

---

36 *American Journal of Nutrition*, 2018, from *TIME Magazine* article

Eat breakfast

Studies show that people who eat whole foods for breakfast tend to have fewer cravings for sweets and make healthier food choices throughout the day. A regular meal pattern that includes breakfast may reduce inflammation and improve quality of sleep. Some women feel that skipping a meal is a good way to cut overall calories, but a recent study showed that skipping breakfast was not a factor in either losing or gaining weight.[37]

Get enough fluids

A good guideline for fluid intake is to divide your body pounds in half and drink that number of fluids in ounces. So, if you weigh 140 pounds, you need about 70 ounces. This amount can include water, juice, milk, tea, etc. Although fruit juice is high in natural sugar, you can try mixing them with vegetable juices or diluting them with water. If your fluid intake includes a lot of soda or diet soda, consider substituting bubbly water with fresh lemon or lime.

Embrace the Mediterranean Diet

It's the best good habit of all, consistently showing a wide range of physical, mental health, and reproductive benefits.[38]

There is no single definition of the Mediterranean Diet, so you don't need to run out and buy a book about it, unless you

37 Sievert, K, "Effect of breakfast on weight and energy intake: systematic review and meta-analysis of randomised controlled trials," *BMJ*. 2019; 364: l42. Published online 2019 Jan 30.

38 Kermack, AJ, "Effect of 6-week 'Mediterranean' dietary intervention on *in vitro* human-embryo development: the Pre-conception Dietary Supplements in Assisted Reproduction double-blinded randomized controlled trial," *Gynecology and Obstetrics*, February 2020 P. 260-269.

want recipes. It is a way of eating that includes lots of fruits and vegetables every day, fish one or two times per week, poultry, beans, eggs, good fats (like olive oil), moderate portions of dairy, and limited red meat. It is not about counting calories, fasting, cutting out major food groups, or never having dessert.

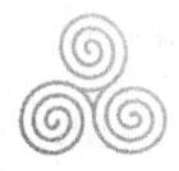

Supplements—snake oil or helpful?

It's hard to eat well all of the time. There's no harm in taking supplements, right?

SUPPLEMENTS ARE AN APPROXIMATELY $30 billion industry, filling up store shelves and constantly popping up online. Their benefit to you depends on whether the supplement contains something you need. Dietary supplements are anything from vitamins and minerals to enzymes, herbs, and protein powders. In an effort to Recover and Renourish, you may have tried various supplements. There are very important supplements, like folic acid, with solid science supporting its use, but for many others, there is not enough solid research to support their safety or efficacy. Frequently, the research that does exist is done by the manufacturers, and the products do not always contain what is printed on the label. In other words, there is a lot of snake oil out there.

Supplementation is not a new idea and has been used for hundreds of years. Back in the 1880s, they were called "tonics" or "elixirs" and were hawked by men who usually left town after the sale. Their bait-and-switch tactics led to the term "snake oil." Snake oil actually does work for the pain of arthritis and bursitis, if it is from the Chinese Erabu water snake, whose oil contained lots of anti-inflammatory Omega-3. Chinese railroad workers shared it with their fellow laborers for joint and muscle pain, but traveling salesmen used rattlesnake and mineral oil, which didn't work, because they lack the Omega-3.

I saw a fertility supplement that is supposed to help egg quality. Should I take it if I want to continue trying to conceive?
Was snake oil listed as the first ingredient? Just kidding. If you could be sure that the supplement was safe and effective, then my answer would be "Yes." But the problem is that, contrary to popular belief, the FDA does not research or approve supplements, and existing research is often done by the manufacturer. The FDA limits the supplement industry by prohibiting claims about specific diseases. Manufacturers are allowed to say vague things like "Enhances Fertility" as opposed to making claims like "Reverses and Cures Ovarian Failure." But there again, no proof is required in regard to a product's ability to "enhance fertility" or even what that means, in order to be on the market. The other thing to consider is if a supplement does, indeed, have hormone-like properties that could affect ovarian function, do you really want to be adding it to any prescribed hormones you may be taking without good research on interactions?

It is understandable that my patient Lexi put herself on extra zinc after reading an article about the possible (but not proven) association between zinc deficiency and poor egg development. She did not have a known zinc deficiency and was already getting zinc in her diet and pre-natal vitamin. Only small amounts of zinc are needed each day, and surpassing the upper limit can interfere with the absorption of another needed micronutrient, copper. Lexi was taking it to help her chances of getting pregnant, but more is not necessarily better when it comes to even "natural" micronutrients like vitamins.

Vitamins and multivitamins have the ingredients and amounts clearly listed on labels for you to check along with how much or how much more than the daily requirement they contain. To further complicate things, manufacturers sometimes add ingredients to supplements and don't list the amounts, considering them a "proprietary blend."

I once called a company to ask about the contents of a proprietary blend of an "adrenal support" supplement. A patient in menopause brought it to my attention because she felt it really decreased her fatigue and hot flashes. The ingredients included bovine adrenal glands, and I really wanted to hear that the ground-up glands were from healthy, happy cows, not the ones sent to the slaughterhouse for spare parts because they were old or ill. The company rep acted as if it were a prank call and was not willing to share any information with me.

What follows is not meant to be a complete list of all fertility supplements you will see on the shelves. These are the supplements my patients frequently ask about or have tried.

Chasteberry, aka vitex (the botanical name), is a bush that grows in Central Asia and the Mediterranean. Consuming its berries was believed to quell sexual desire and so was used by celibate monks, hence the common name, chasteberry. The linoleic acid in the berry binds to estrogen-receptor cells, which are located throughout the reproductive system. This quality is perhaps part of the connection to potential hormonal effects.

This is speculation on my part, but, perhaps, when the monks ate the "estrogenic" berries, it lowered their testosterone (which estrogen can do), resulting in decreased libido.

There is some research indicating that supplements containing vitex may increase mid-cycle progesterone levels (the number of days after ovulation or the luteal phase), resulting in a longer luteal phase and higher pregnancy rates.

Anecdotally, some of my patients have reported that their short luteal phase lengthened after taking vitex for a few months, but this did not happen for others. If you want to try it, check with your doctor first, and try to make sure you have ovulated for that cycle, as there is some literature indicating chasteberry can delay ovulation.

The bottom line is that vitex does have a hormonal effect, but exactly what it does or how it will react with your own hormones is not precisely known. For that reason, women are advised against taking it when on any kind of hormonal therapy including birth-control pills or if they have hormone-sensitive conditions like breast cancer. If you decide to try vitex, have a clear vision of what it is you are trying to accomplish (e.g., a longer luteal phase, less spotting before full flow, or relief from hot flashes), and then carefully set benchmarks that you track. If you do not see a change, do not continue taking it. The length of a trial period is not something I can state with authority, but two or three months is probably reasonable.

Maca-Maca. This starchy vegetable from the cauliflower, broccoli, kale, and cabbage family, looks a bit like a turnip and grows in Peru. The roots are ground into a powder and marketed as a fertility supplement. While there is some research to show that it can lower blood pressure and improve mood when compared to a placebo, there is no conclusive research proving its effects on hormonal balance and fertility. Research that I reviewed involved comparing maca to a placebo, but not to an increased intake of other types of vegetable roots. I suspect it might not necessarily prove to be superior to an increased intake of other high-quality vegetables from the same family.

L-arginine. This is an amino acid that is a building block for protein. It is made in the body and plays a role in the immune system and in the synthesis of nitric oxide, a blood gas involved in many physiological processes, including vasodilation. It has been studied for its effects on both male and female fertility. In theory, vasodilation will result in better blood flow to organs, which, in turn, leads to better organ function. But how this plays out with reproductive organs is not conclusive. Know that supplementation can trigger outbreaks of the herpes virus because arginine is key to the replication of herpes simplex in the body. Good dietary sources for L-arginine are nuts, seeds, oats, corn, buckwheat, brown rice, dairy, meat, and dark chocolate.

L-carnitine. This is also an amino acid that acts an antioxidant, helping with energy production and metabolism. It is an important antioxidant, meaning it helps the body get rid of the waste products of cells. These qualities may be the reason it has shown promise in fertility—when all your cells are getting the energy they need and the waste products removed, your general health and, therefore, reproductive health for men and women may be enhanced.[39] There are positive and negative studies on whether L-carnitine improves sperm quality.

Your body makes L-arginine and L-carnitine, but eating nuts, seeds, peas, beans, dairy products, fish, and meat (in moderation) is a good way to ensure you get the building blocks for them. If you are vegetarian, asparagus and whole grains are good sources.

CoQ10. Coenzyme Q10 is a vitamin-like substance that is present in every organ. It has an important supporting role in cell division.

Because CoQ10 is a player in cell division and metabolism, it has worked its way into the fertility-care toolbox. You know what is coming next: not enough research to draw broad conclusions regarding reproductive health. It is considered safe to take within the suggested dose ranges. If you are considering conception in the future, some proponents believe that you need to take CoQ10 for about four months for it to work its way into your cell physiology. Because CoQ10 is needed by all muscles, including the heart, it has become a popular supplement.

Myo-Inositol. A member of the vitamin B family, it is sometimes referred to as B8. It is made by the body, and, therefore, in theory, you don't need to take a supplement. Researchers thought that taking it *might* enhance egg quality because poor-quality eggs were found to have low levels of myo-inositol in the fluid around them. However, there is good evidence that myo-inositol and its cousins are helpful only in situations where a woman has insulin resistance, which occurs in pre-diabetes and PCOS or polycystic ovarian syndrome. In this case, myo-inositol may help the body use insulin better, facilitating ovulation and more

39 Agarwal, A, "Role of L-carnitine in Female Infertility," *Reproductive Biology and Endocrinology*, 2018.

regular menstrual cycles. Supplemental myo-inositol is considered safe when recommended amounts are not exceeded, but get direction from your doctor if you choose to take it. Myo-inositol in its natural form is found in lima beans, navy beans, oranges, grapefruit, cantaloupe, grains, and nuts.

DHEA. DHEA is an abbreviation for dehydroepiandrosterone. Not to be confused with DHA, which is a valuable omega-3 fatty acid. That's 22 letters. I could start by recommending that you should never take a supplement with that many letters, but there would be no scientific basis for me to say that. DHEA is an endogenous (already in our body) substance produced in the adrenal glands that helps produce testosterone and other hormones. It has been studied in relation to its possible positive effects on osteoporosis, depression, and vaginal atrophy, but no solid conclusions can be drawn from the literature. There is some research indicating that women with lower levels of DHEA might benefit from supplementation in terms of the number of retrieved eggs in IVF, clinical pregnancy rate, and live birth.[40] Some researchers have also looked at the possible positive benefits on uterine endometrial lining. DHEA may help women with poor egg quality, so some doctors recommend it. Because DHEA is essentially a precursor to hormones and many of my patients are already on hormone supplementation, I strongly encourage women to have a discussion with their doctor before taking it. If you decide to put yourself on it, consider the recommendation from many doctors that you take it for a limited time, not indefinitely.

Melatonin. This is an example of another supplement *not* to take just because you read testimonials on a website or in a

---

40 *Ibid.*

chatroom. There is scientific evidence that this naturally-occurring and powerful antioxidant hormone increases egg and embryo quality in those little creatures we trap with cheese, but limited evidence for this effect in humans. Here is the caveat: exogenous (from outside the body) melatonin may confuse a woman's hormones and disrupt her menstrual cycles. This is not a concern when a woman's cycles are controlled by IVF medications, but melatonin is probably not a good idea if you will be trying to conceive naturally.

Royal Jelly. I don't get asked about this as often as I did several years ago (supplements trend in cycles), but mythology persists surrounding this wonderful natural substance. A Queen Bee can lay up to 60,000 eggs per day when she dines on the royal jelly that the worker bees make fresh for her every day. Unfortunately, the active ingredient in royal jelly responsible for this egg-producing effect becomes inactive several hours after production. If you have been eating royal jelly, you did get some nice B vitamins, but probably it's not reason enough to eat a lot of very expensive peanut butter and royal jelly sandwiches.

I am not anti-supplement. I just want to protect you from snake oil, substituting supplements for whole food, and taking something that is contraindicated with your prescribed meds. It is vital that you check with your doctor about supplements and stick with their recommendations or vetoes. But he or she cannot be expected to be knowledgeable about the hundreds of products on the market, as well as the exponential number of interactions. I wanted this book to have a long shelf life, but the other thing to know about supplements is that future research may outdate information here or in other books.

My patient Rachel had done a lot of reading about supplements and really wanted to try a lot of them. Her doctor was not convinced of their safety and efficacy for her low ovarian reserve, and this was disappointing to her. What was ultimately the best route for Rachel was to find a doctor who was all in on supplementation and had a "Well, it probably won't hurt you" approach. Fortunately, a number of researchers are keeping track of whether certain supplements enhance fertility. Stay tuned. I'll update this information in my blog.

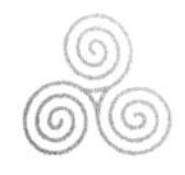

Eating for happiness

I tried so hard to eat well and take the right supplements for so long, and I still don't have a baby. I'm tired of trying. How do I get out of this slump?

BY GETTING BACK INTO EATING FOR PLEASURE and not just for weight loss, hormonal balance, or procreation.

Now that you know how to eat for health and healing, I want to inspire you to enjoy eating, to eat for happiness. Your journey to start a family has had some unhappy moments, and you deserve to be happy. Food can help. We have all discovered our comfort foods for good reason. We are biologically programmed to enjoy food, as evidenced by the reward system that lights up in our brain when we eat. Lactose, the sugar found in breast milk, is sweet to the taste and keeps babies coming back for more.

If you believe that happiness is, in part, the absence of depression, anxiety, and the inability to enjoy life, you will be impressed with the research on food and mood. Felice

Jacka, PhD, nutritionist and pioneer in the new field of Nutritional Psychiatry, studied 67 people with moderate to severe anxiety who were eating an unhealthy diet. Half the group were enrolled in nutrition counseling in which they were encouraged to eat a diet high in fruits, vegetables, grains, and fish—basically the Mediterranean Diet. The other half were treated with "social support," which involved giving them opportunities for friendly conversation, with no dietary intervention. After 12 weeks, about 30% of those who received dietary support were in remission from their depression compared to only 8% in the social-support group.[41]

Scientists devoted to the study of nutrition and mental health believe that the brain needs folate, the omega-3 fatty acids EPA and DHA, vitamins A and C, the B vitamins, including thiamine (also known as B1), and the minerals iron, selenium, and zinc to regulate mood and prevent depression. Foods high in these nutrients include fish and shellfish, like clams, mussels, and oysters. Plant foods that are high in these nutrients include leafy greens, colorful peppers, broccoli, and cauliflower. Instead of trying to make mental notes on these nutrients and foods that have them, just eat five to seven servings of colorful fruits and vegetables every day, some seafood each week, high-quality grains, and high-quality fats to help you absorb the nutrients, and you will have covered the bases. Eating this way is associated with less risk of anxiety and depression.[42]

---

41 Jacka, F, *Brain Changer: The Good Mental Health Diet*. February 2019, Macmillan.

42 Liu, X, "Fruit and vegetable consumption and the risk of depression: A meta-analysis," *Nutrition*. 2016 Mar;32(3):296-302.

I have heard that some people's problem with mood may be related to their intestines. How is that possible?
You heard right. Many of the neurotransmitters your brain needs, such as the "feel-good chemical" serotonin, are produced in your gut. Your intestines need to be healthy and functioning well with the proper amounts of good bacteria on hand to produce neurotransmitters. These healthy bacteria, known as the microbiome, have an important role in immune-system function and in the extraction of energy from food. This is the reason for the popularity of taking probiotics, which can increase good bacteria. But as with all supplements, they might not be needed, and they don't necessarily work preventively. In other words, if your lawn is already thick and green, you don't need fertilizer. There is some evidence that a good microbiome is enhanced by fermented foods such as kefir, unsweetened yogurt, and sauerkraut.

My approach to "eating for happiness" can be summed up as, *Everything in moderation, even moderation.* In other words, if you want to enjoy an occasional piece of chocolate cake, cookie, or ice cream cone, and it makes you happy, please do that. Eat it mindfully, savoring every bite without guilt. Just don't have a second piece. Or save half of the super-sized muffins and giant cookies commonly sold in bakeries for another day. I know—they get stale. But freeze them. And be sure to eat six or more servings of fruits and vegetables every day. I know I have repeated this last guideline several times so far. It's because it is that important.

OK, now that you've told me I can enjoy chocolate cake, I am inspired to eat well again. I have seen lists of "Super Foods." What are they?

There are no special "super foods." Eating a variety of high-quality protein, carbohydrate, and fats will nourish you well enough to be considered "super foods." In addition to these macronutrients, your five to seven servings of fruits and vegetables that I keep harping about will provide the vitamins and minerals you need for health and healing. I should remind you that some scientists and nutritionists advise that people eat even more than five to seven servings per day. If you feel that, as much as you try, you are not eating well enough, a multivitamin is a good idea—and one with folic acid if you will be trying to conceive. There is solid research that the folic-acid status of the father is as important as the mother's because of its effect on the quality of embryos.[43]

If you would feel more inspired by having a list of specific foods to zero in on for health and healing, here are some I recommend: eggs (organic), avocados, kale, kiwi, beans, cilantro, olive oil, blueberries, apples, quinoa, walnuts, almonds, salmon, and cod. At the risk of adding controversy, I am going to put organic milk on my list, and not just because my dear friends Kim and Darrell are dairy farmers. Vitamin-fortified organic milk is a good source of vitamin D, calcium, and protein. Two percent or whole milk will provide more of the fat you need as opposed to skim milk, but if you prefer it and are getting fat from other sources, that is okay.

In addition to lists of Super Foods, you have probably seen lists of "Foods for Fertility." Pineapple is trending right now, to

---

43 Hoek, J, "Does the father matter? The association between the peri-conceptional paternal folate status and embryonic growth." *Fertility and Sterility* Feb. 2016, pp. 270–277

the point where pineapples have become a symbol (available on lapel pins and jewelry) of fertility struggles and hopes. Pineapple is considered a fertility food in Traditional Chinese Medicine, where it was prescribed to "keep blood flowing in the palace for the baby," aka the uterus. This is where fact, fact, and a leap of logic come into play. Fact: pineapple contains bromelain, which is a natural blood thinner because it reduces clotting time and, in effect, keeps the blood flowing. Fact: clotting of tiny blood vessels would theoretically be harmful to a developing baby. My leap: eating pineapple may prevent the harmful clotting that might cause failure of an embryo to implant or thrive.

Fast-forward to modern medicine, in which some women with repeat pregnancy loss are sometimes found to have certain antibodies associated with inflammation and blood-clotting tendencies. Known as anti-phospholipid antibody disorder, it is treated with medications to "thin" the blood and reduce the chances of clotting to see if it helps a woman avoid another miscarriage.

Whether or not the bromelain in the pineapple can thin blood, consuming it does not have a downside. Although, now that I think about it, it did have a downside for one patient, years ago. I mentioned that she should enjoy some pineapple, given her history of unexplained miscarriages, and she came to her next visit with sores all over the inside of her mouth and lips because she had eaten a large amount of this acidic fruit. You can understand the desire to do all that you can to conceive. I learned to be much more specific after that, and I recommend just one serving (about one cup) of pineapple or ½ cup of pineapple core per day. The core contains more bromelain than the fruit, but it is tough, fibrous, and flavorless, so if you pass on it, it's understandable.

Traditional Chinese Medicine believes certain foods can enhance a person's fertility by building "Yin." These foods include asparagus, raspberries, string beans, sweet potatoes, pumpkin and squashes, shellfish, oysters, and eggs.

Is it true that something called "seed cycling" can help painful periods, hot flashes, and fertility?

Seed cycling for hormonal balance and fertility is trending right now and may have some potential. "Seed cycling" calls for eating ground flax, pumpkin, sesame, and sunflower seeds at different times in the menstrual cycle. Seeds may have some hormonal benefits because they are high in lignans, a substance with weakly estrogenic and anti-estrogenic properties. A study in the *Journal of Endocrinology Metabolism* indicated that consumption of flaxseed powder resulted in a longer luteal phase,[44] but much of the evidence is anecdotal. Patients have told me that they experienced less painful and more regular cycles after seed cycling for about three months, and some perimenopausal women have experienced reduced symptoms. If you want to try seed cycling, it seems safe, and seeds have many good micronutrients. There is ample information on the types, amounts, and rotation of seeds available online (Google Seed Cycling), but do remember to grind only about a week's worth at a time and store the ground and unground seeds in the refrigerator, as seeds become rancid after about three months. I am not convinced that there is enough evidence to warrant a specific schedule for when each seed type is consumed in a cycle, so I tell my patients it is okay to just put ground seeds

---

44 Phipps, WR, "Effect of flax seed ingestion on the menstrual cycle," *J Clin Endocrinal Metab.* 1993 Nov;77(5):1215-9

in their smoothies, soups, or salads on a regular basis. Grinding the seeds is necessary to release the helpful component, lignans.

I know I should lose weight whether I will be conceiving or not. Should I see a dietician or a nutritionist? I don't even know the difference.

Yes, a consultation with a skilled dietician or nutritionist could definitely help. But like choosing a doctor or plumber, you want to pick a skilled one.

A dietician is a nutrition and food expert whose background includes the science of food and its effect on health. They must pass stringent exams and become a registered and licensed dietician (RD) to practice. Many work in hospitals and clinics where they manage the nutrition therapy for specific diseases like diabetes and cancer.

The title "nutritionist" is used by people with a broad range of training and credentials. Some states require that nutritionists be certified as a nutrition specialist (CNS designation) to use the title, but in many states, credentialing and licensing are not required, and anyone may call themselves a "nutritionist," "nutrition coach," or "nutrition counselor." I have met hospital-based dieticians who seem to still be using a food pyramid from decades ago. I have also encountered nutritionists who think that the answer to everything is to eat another supplement. The bottom line is to check credentials and the experience of practitioners you are considering.

I hear what you are saying about how tiring it is to figure out the right things to eat. This could become easier to figure out in the future owing to the evolving sciences of nutrigenomics and nutrigenetics. Nutrigenomics is the study of how different foods interact with your particular genome (your 3 billion base pairs of DNA that make up your chromosomes) while nutrigenetics aims to determine how people will respond to specific nutrients. This information may someday help you choose the right foods for your digestive system and perhaps avoid the expression of genes that cause diseases like Celiac and Crohn's.

Someday it may be possible to really refine which fruits and vegetables are best for an individual and which will not be readily absorbed and utilized. Being handed a list of foods scientifically proven to either help or harm you based on your DNA may be a relief on one hand, but it will not be great for me if chocolate-chip cookies are on my *Do Not Eat* list. These two new sciences are so exciting that I would like to be a nutrigeneticist in my next life, but I will have to come back with a much higher IQ.

Patients sometimes bring in results of tests of blood and saliva done by companies claiming to know which foods a person should never eat based on an "allergic" response. Be careful: Many of these companies are dealing in pseudo-science and do not have adequate research to support their testing methods and advice. While the clinical application of nutrigenomics and nutrigenetics is exciting to think about, more research is needed to clinically apply these evolving sciences.

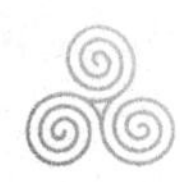

Revitalizing the Physical You

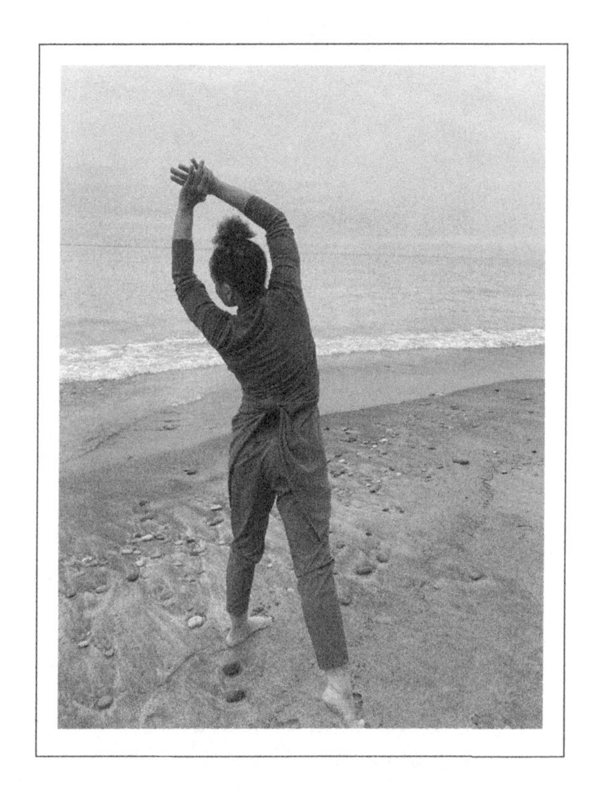

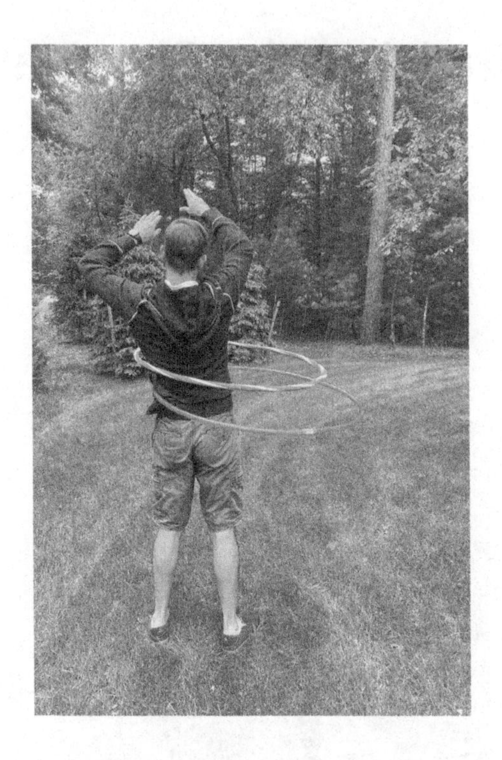

Research shows that hula hooping
with weighted hoops burns
calories, tones abdominal muscles,
and lowers bad cholesterol.

A conversation over tea

Peppermint Tea Peppermint and spearmint plants are members of the *menthe* genus, whose leaves make a cooling and aromatic tea that can reduce nasal congestion, cough, and nausea. The cooling properties of peppermint make it a logical choice if one is a bit overheated after playing or working out.

A substance known as *menthe* in peppermint oil activates cold-sensitive receptors in the skin and mucosal tissues, which accounts for the cooling sensation.

Getting back to "normal"

WHEN PATIENTS SHARE THEIR GOALS about "getting back to normal," they often include losing weight and gaining energy, both good steps toward Revitalization.

You have spent a lot of time and energy trying to eat the right foods, lower your stress, and stay in shape physically in an effort to conceive and have a healthy pregnancy. Maybe you didn't always stay on track, but, for the most part, you tried hard and did well. But you still may have ended up feeling physically depleted after months of hormone supplementation, induced periods, heavy periods, miscarriage, or a difficult pregnancy.

I'm not even sure if I want to keep trying to have a baby. I just want to lose the weight I've gained over these last months. What exercise will be the fastest way?
Let's talk about the *best* way, not just the fastest way.

I have seen many patients push themselves to jog, do interval classes, lift weights, spin, and hot yoga in an effort to get back on track physically or lose weight. While these activities are not inherently bad, they can drain rather than Revitalize if you are already depleted. I advocate a gentler approach to fitness that will potentially be more sustainable and nourishing.

Sometimes the amount of weight a person wants to lose seems overwhelming. For many of my patients, signs of ovarian function and regular periods returned after losing some, but not all, the weight they wanted to lose.

Losing weight, in most cases, can be accomplished by simply eating less and moving more. A person can lose weight with doing just one of these two things, but the combination is the best strategy. Changing eating and activity habits takes time and commitment, so be patient with yourself. A non-judgmental attitude about your body size and shape is the best mindset when trying to lose weight. Fat-shaming yourself is not productive.

Instead of focusing on weight and shape, it can be helpful to think about physical vitality and what vitality feels like to you. If you are doing challenging exercise classes, don't jump on the scale afterward. Instead, ask yourself, *Do I feel energized, stronger, Revitalized?* It is normal to feel "spent" after vigorous exercise, but if fatigue or low energy occur, you may be draining your basic body energy (known as *Qi* in Eastern medicine). Remember the words of Lao Tzu: "Better to stop short than to fill to the brim . . . Oversharpen the blade, and the edge will soon blunt."

If you have an exercise routine but still feel overweight and have low energy or if you have not found a physical activity you can stick with, consider inspiring yourself by moving in new and different ways.

You probably know about the excellent cardiovascular and strength-building benefits of running, yoga, weightlifting, etc. I don't want to take up your time to by talking about those usual sorts of activities you probably have tried or do regularly. If you have an exercise routine you like, stay with it, but if you want to expand your horizon or have not found an activity that you like, let's keep talking.

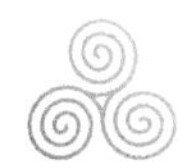

Couch potato or tomato?

How do I know if I need to push myself to be more active, or let up a bit?

TO ANSWER THAT, LET'S LOOK AT THE EXTREMES, because I want you to be in the middle. You don't want to be a couch potato; you want to be a couch tomato.

"Couch potato" is a term often used to describe someone who is inactive and sits around a lot. Potatoes are a much-maligned vegetable. They are high in vitamins C and B6 but are associated with being starchy, dry, bumpy, and stored in warehouses for long periods of time. An esoteric plant-biology-journal author described potatoes as having "low metabolic activity."

Tomatoes, on the other hand, are described by botanists as having "dramatic metabolic changes during development." They start out green, ripen to a smooth red skin, and are loaded with moist seeds inside, which makes them, botanically, a fruit. As you try to heal and regain your physical vitality, I want you to think of yourself as a couch tomato, meaning I want you to be physically and metabolically active, moist inside, and smooth skinned. But I want you to rest on a couch as needed. You have been through a lot, and good-quality sleep and rest are key to recovery, not exercising yourself into exhaustion.

I am a runner, not a couch potato, so I'm good, right?
That depends on how much you are running. Many of my patients are committed to running, Pilates, Barre, hot yoga, and power yoga. However, there is a downside to some of these types of activities. Excessive running can be hard on joints and the spine. But my main concern for you is that excessive exercise can deplete your body of fat and burn up the fat you eat. This, in turn, can compromise your ability to rebuild hormones since fat is the main component of estrogen and progesterone. If you are trying to lose weight by running, remember that the more you run, the more efficient your muscles become, in which case, you will burn fewer calories. If you really like to run and will be going through ovarian stimulation, check with your doctor on the recommended limit of miles per week.

I really have put on a lot of fat around my stomach. I'm not that vain, but I hate the way it looks. What can I do?
I hear women criticizing their abdomens frequently. I know that jeans can feel a bit tight during hormone supplementation or early pregnancy, but I think sometimes patients have a distorted view of what their abdomen looks like.

A lovely Hmong woman of normal weight came to me a few years ago after three failed embryo transfers. I noticed that she was wearing a very tight girdle, like something from the 1950s.

She wore it most of the time, she said, so that her husband "would not see my fat stomach." I convinced her to stop wearing the girdle so that her *Qi* and blood could flow more freely to and from the "palace for the baby" during her next IVF. Wonderfully, she had a healthy baby boy nine months after this fourth transfer. Although I cannot say for sure that reducing external abdominal restriction and acupuncture enhanced her *Qi* and blood flow to the uterus, it is known in Western *and* Traditional Chinese Medicine that good blood flow to reproductive organs is necessary for a successful pregnancy.

Whether a woman's view of her body shape is distorted or accurate, a self-image of tummy fat can make a woman eager to work on strengthening her abs. Be kind and accepting of your abdomen, so as not to complicate healing. There is a situation known as *diastasis recti*, which is a stretching of the abdominal muscles where they meet mid-abdomen. This stretching is a normal and necessary function that allows the abdomen to expand for a growing baby. However, sometimes after a delivery, the tissues connecting the muscles do not pull together tightly, and the belly will seem less flat. Know if you have this that certain exercises such as crunches, planks, and twists can make the separation worse. Plus, too many or improperly done sit-ups and crunches will put downward pressure on the pelvic-floor muscles, which hold the uterus, rectum, and bladder in place, eventually weakening rather than strengthening them. Pelvic-floor weakness is a common problem that happens not overnight but over time—just look at the huge amount of shelf space for adult diapers in the store. Please try to avoid walking down that aisle by taking care of yourself now.

In the spirit of exploring new ways of moving and to answer your question about tummy fat, I must tell you about my competitive hula-hooping patient, Alexis. I was indeed intrigued by her vocation, which involved traveling to hula-hoop tournaments and performing in parks with hoops, some of which were on fire. The first time I tried to insert my sterile, hair-thin (but sharp) needles two inches on either side of her belly button, the needle just slowly curved and would not go in. Her slim waist was comprised of abdominal muscles that were beyond taut. As it turns out, there is good research showing that hula hooping with a weighted hoop burns calories, tones abdominal muscles, and lowers bad cholesterol. In one study, participants lost 1.34 inches from their waist in six weeks. You don't need much space; you can learn via YouTube.

What do you think about hot yoga for shaping up?

I get asked this a lot, because it has become so popular. As a Witch Doctor, I believe that hot yoga is an oxymoron, meaning that only morons do it. *Just kidding.* In my opinion, yoga is about balance and union, not extremes of hot or cold.

Hot yoga can raise your internal body temperature. We are designed to function best at about 98.6 degrees. While some say a 100-degree room allows them to stretch their muscles more, overstretching can cause injuries. Intense sweating can be unhealthy as well, as it can lead to dehydration.

In Traditional Chinese Medicine, we believe that too much sweating drains a woman's "Yin," which is necessary for reproductive energy. I truly believe that hot yoga may have a bit of an addictive property—some of my patients have rejected my advice to discontinue it, even though they truly want to conceive.

I tell them about Shannon, a woman who was not trying to conceive but was entering menopause. She came to me for help with severe, unremitting hot flashes. We noticed a definite pattern of relief from her hot flashes when she went on vacation and stopped going to hot-yoga classes five times a week. Hot flashes occur because of the effect of hormones on blood vessels. In pre-menopause, hormone levels are roller-coasting around. I wondered if the frequent hot yoga was stressing her dwindling supply of hormones. Again, this is my *fact, fact, and leap* way of thinking (common to Witch Doctors) when pondering a clinical question. It is a fact that she was having severe hot flashes, and a fact that they stopped when she stopped hot yoga. What the exact relationship is between hot yoga and its possible effect on hormone balance is not clear from this anecdote, but my opinion is that "regular" yoga is safer if you are trying to enhance your hormonal balance. Hopefully I did not offend my hot-yoga-instructor patients with my "moron" joke. I believe hot yoga is probably okay if you are not trying to conceive.

I am not aware of any cold-yoga classes, but Wim Hof, a Dutch extreme athlete, has made a name for himself by sitting naked in piles of snow for long periods of time in order to boost his immune system. He holds the Guinness record for swimming under ice and has won a half-marathon barefoot in snow. I wouldn't be surprised if cold-yoga classes appear on the scene someday, but don't take them.

Power yoga can also be a contradiction in terms if you push yourself hard to keep up with too many non-stop sun salutations or headstands. What I call *regular yoga* and some call *Hatha yoga* would be my choice for you as you Revitalize.

I guess I can cool it on the sit-ups, running, and hot yoga, but what am I supposed to do then?
Walk.

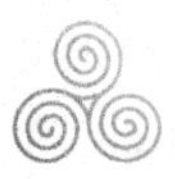

In praise of walking

In Praise of Walking is a book, by neuroscientist Shaun O'Mara, that presents the science of how walking strengthens muscles and bones, improves brain function and mood, and "inoculates against depression and fosters creativity." It seems incontrovertible that as Hippocrates said, "Walking is the best medicine," but sometimes we need evidence-based appeals to inspire us to adopt behaviors. Thank you, Dr. O'Mara—your book provides that.

Walking, along with other types of movement, stimulates the growth of new cells in the hippocampus, the area of the brain involved with memory and learning. In addition to this, vascular endothelial growth factor (VEGF), which promotes the growth of tiny blood vessels, is activated by walking. Brain plasticity, the ability of brain neurons to grow and reorganize, is another body process markedly enhanced by walking.

New news may be the effect of walking on *creativity.* While difficult to measure, the research of Dr. Christian Rominger has shown a positive association between walking and improved creativity.[45]

Many of my patients tell me that, between work and doctor's appointments, it is difficult to attend scheduled exercise classes. There certainly is an abundance of exercise classes online, but, once again, the challenge is finding the time to do them. One of the most accessible forms of exercise is walking, because we can insert it into our daily schedule.

Our ancestors had to traverse many miles in search of dinner and walk the fields to gather grain. People walked a lot until the invention of wheels—then motorized cars and then TV. Walking to school, work, or the grocery store is not part of daily life for most of us. We need to look for opportunities to walk consistently, because, in addition to the brain and muscle benefits, it is one of the most effective ways to lose weight. Brisk walking is more effective than slow walking, and steps really do add up, as you may know if you have played with a fitness tracker. If you don't seem to be getting close to the recommended 10,000 steps a day, make a habit of taking the stairs instead of elevators or escalators, and park your car in the far corner of a store lot. Do this all of the time, not just when the weather is good. Ideally, walking briskly 30 minutes, four or five times per week, is a great start. If this is not possible, try to reserve ten minutes, or more, of your lunch hour for a brisk walk outside or around your office building. Outside

---

45 Rominger, C, "Everyday bodily movement is associated with creativity independently from active positive affect: a Bayesian mediation-analysis approach, *Sci Rep* 10, 11985 (2020)

walking shows more benefits, possibly because it may incorporate opportunities to commune with the healing powers of nature. If you don't get a lunch hour, work on that as step one. Short walks will add up to an impressive number, not unlike small purchases on your credit card. One fitness expert has claimed that 15,000 steps is the new 10,000, but just start with an easier goal.

The ability to socialize while walking should move walking to the top of your activity list. For busy people, it's a brilliant way to keep in touch with friends, ideally in person, but if necessary, also while on the phone.

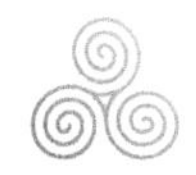

Get in touch with your inner crane

ANOTHER WAY TO EXPLORE MOVEMENT is to get in touch with your inner crane, bear, monkey, tiger, or deer. This advice comes to us from the ancients, who didn't have tennis clubs, golf courses, or gyms available to them. But they understood the importance of movement and looked to their natural environment to see what would be helpful. What they saw were cranes, bears, tigers, and monkeys, moving in interesting and athletic ways. Practicing these animal movements for physical conditioning, coordination, and mind-body balance was credited to Chinese physician Hua Tuo (208-145 BC) and were known as "The Five Frolics."[46] These animal-inspired movements evolved into a form of martial art called *Tai Qi* or *Tai Chi*. From a Western point of view, the movements improve postural balance and mental

46 Garofalo, MP, "Animal Frolics. An Ancient Chinese Exercise Regimen for Nourishing Life," available online https://www.egreenway.com/qigong/animalfrolics.htm

focus. *Tai Qi* can help a person relax, sleep better, and possibly lower blood pressure.[47,48]

If you want to spend more time meditating but have found it difficult to sit still on a cushion and quiet your mind, focusing on the sequence of movements in *Tai Qi* feels like a moving form of mindful meditation.

"*Tai Qi* and *Qi Gong* practices include a mindfulness component, which may explain why some patients experience greater benefits from *Tai Qi* or *Qi Gong* than from general aerobic exercises."[49]

Isn't Tai Qi for old people?

I am sure that is what the young Chinese medical students were thinking as they stared and giggled at my class in Guangzhou, China.

It was common in China to see older people imitating a crane while waiting for a bus, but I never saw young people practicing. Maybe things have changed—I was there years ago, during my internship. Because most of the research has focused on whether *Tai Qi* can decrease falls and frailty in the elderly, it is viewed as an activity for seniors. Many of you have asked me for help with sleep, blood pressure, and sense of well-being, which practicing *Tai Qi* can improve. I am not aware of any data indicating that the benefits of *Tai Qi* are age-specific, so keep an open mind.

Qi (meaning "breath") and *Gong* (meaning "work") is another form of movement with healing and Revitalizing benefits. Like

47 Huston, P, "Health Benefits of *Tai Qi*. What Is the Evidence?" 2014 *Can Fam Physician* 2016 Nov;62(11):881-890.

48 "*Tai Qi* for your Health: A Modern Take on an Ancient Practice," https://newsinhealth.nih.gov/2016/12/tai-chi-your-health

49 https://www.ncbi.nlm.nih.gov/pmc/articles/PMC3917559/

Tai Qi, *Qi Gong* is believed to increase the "life force" that every organ needs. The idea that this breath or energy is key to health was not only a Chinese concept. Eastern Indians called it *prana*, the Japanese, *ki*, the Greeks, *pneuma*, and the Hebrews, *ruah*. Modern scientists trying to measure this life force often describe it in terms of atoms moving around constantly and predictably in everything.

I found *Qi Gong* much easier to learn because the movements are simpler than *Tai Qi* and are repeated several times before moving on to another. In Eastern Medicine, *Qi Gong* is considered more "medically oriented" because it targets specific types of energy flow to specific organs.

Although a live class offers the advantage of personal guidance, there are hundreds *Tai Qi* and *Qi Gong* videos available on the internet. Be aware that some of the practitioners online make a lot of unsubstantiated claims. One acupuncturist on YouTube chirps into the camera that *Qi Gong* "will stimulate your pituitary, hypothalamus, and thyroid, and help egg formation, implantation, and the uterine lining." There is no research to support these claims.

Also, be wary of "*Qi Gong* Masters," who claim that they can manipulate and touch your body in ways that will help you heal or become more fertile. Scientific evidence is lacking, but if you ever want to try these interventions on the theory that "It can't hurt," make sure that you have thoroughly checked out the person's methods and reputation. A personal testimonial from someone you trust is important. As part of my research into things my patients try, I once went to a *Qi Gong* healer to see what it would be like. I went to a tiny white row house in Milwaukee and laid on a cat-stained carpet as an older man moved his hands gently above my body. I have a vague remembrance that the problem I sought help for slightly improved. It was weird, but I felt safe.

An in-person class is ideal, but if you can't find one near you, I would recommend trying DVDs or online classes. There are an overwhelming number of classes available online. If you don't want to spend time sifting through all of them, Kathy Lang, Helen Liang, Janice Tucker, and Mimi Kuo-Deemer are calm, skilled teachers who communicate well. Just Google their names, followed by the words *Tai Qi* and *Qi Gong*, and their videos and websites will come up. Beginning levels are often free, with reasonable fees for continuing.

Although there is not enough research to prove the benefits to reproductive health of *Tai Qi* and *Qi Gong*, I believe the gentle, breath-based, and meditative movements of *Tai Qi* and *Qi Gong* counterbalance the clenching, flexing, and tightening movements that characterize current popular exercises like Barre, Pilates, and kettlebells.

If you prefer books over videos, *Qi Gong for Fertility Enhancement*, by Dr. Randine Lewis, is an excellent source of information. *The Tao of Fertility*, by Dr. Daoshing Ni, has good illustrations and instructions on *Qi Gong* for pelvic and reproductive health.

Okay. I get that I need to move to feel better, but flapping like a crane is not going to help me lose weight, right?

Right—it probably won't burn a lot of calories.

This gets back to the *calories out must be more than calories in* formula for weight loss. You can do that by eating less or moving more. As we talked about a few minutes ago, doing both will speed up the loss. Try not to get hung up on calories, but be aware of your intake. If you don't have time to exercise on a given day, choose not to have a second cookie, or eat only the bottom bun with your burger. If you really want to eat that ice cream, add some minutes to your treadmill time. This is how food intake and activity work together in its simplest form. If you need an accurate picture of what your calorie intake and output are, there are many tracking apps available. I would recommend trying them with a goal of weaning off them when you get an idea of your pattern. Some people will stay on track better if they use an app indefinitely, but I would love to see you just enjoy food and movement without the risk of hyper-focusing.

Trying new exercises presents the same problems as old exercises. How do I find the time?

You don't find time; you make time.

Lack of time is the reason many of us cite for not being more active. You can't put more hours in the day or days in the week. But have you noticed that we usually find the time to do the things that we really want to do? Think about how you spend your time. Those activities are obviously your priorities—perhaps watching movies, shopping, crafting, baking, reading, blogging, catching up with friends online. There's nothing wrong with those activities, but there are only so many waking hours in the day. The solution to making more time is to switch your mindset, habits, and priorities. If your usual wind-down after work involves watching reruns of *Friends* or online shopping, maybe go for a brisk walk first, even if just for ten minutes, and then watch TV. If you can, walk outside where you can observe trees, sky, bird calls; it is a form of mindful meditation. If catching up with a friend by phone or listening to music while you walk gets you going, that's great. Just please be aware of traffic at crosswalks.

If your workday ends with pickup at daycare, followed by dinner, bath, bedtime stories, and homework help, it goes without saying that these must remain priorities. However, trading nights with your partner or a fellow parent to give you each a free night for self-care is something to consider. I am really impressed with people who can simply get up a bit earlier or go to bed later to make the time to meditate or exercise. I find that very hard to do, but this is where forming new habits and reshuffling priorities comes in.

What you really want to avoid is being sedentary. You are sedentary if you spend most of your day sitting at a computer, in your car, at meetings, followed by reading or watching TV on your sofa. "Sitting is like the new smoking" in terms of cardiovascular risks, according to Mayo Clinic endocrinologist James Levine. Tom Roth, author of *Eat, Move, Sleep*, says "Sitting is the most underrated health threat of modern time." According to some data, the benefits of going to the gym for an hour a day may be reduced by sitting for the rest of the day. A study presented at a 2015 American College of Cardiology meeting showed that regular exercisers had the same buildup of coronary artery calcium (an indicator of heart disease) in their vessels as non-exercisers if they sat for extended periods of time after their workout.[50]

50 Kulinski, J, "Study Bolsters Link Between Heart Disease, Excessive Sitting." https://www.acc.org/about-acc/press-releases/2015/03/05/16/19/study-bolsters-link-between-heart-disease-excessive-sitting

We can't draw too many broad conclusions from this data, but Dr. Jacqueline Kulinski, assistant professor of cardiovascular medicine at The Medical College of Wisconsin, sums it up well: "This study suggests that reducing how much you sit every day may represent a more novel strategy (in addition to exercise) to help reduce your cardiovascular risk."

I am just trying to lose weight and get my hormones balanced again. At age 38, I don't need to be concerned about all this cardiology stuff, do I?

Being sedentary is associated with infertility, type-2 diabetes, and high blood pressure.[51] The buildup of cholesterol and calcium in your arteries doesn't happen overnight. It may be accelerated as we age, but it starts when you are younger.

I have to work at a computer all day, and then I drive to the gym. Are you telling me that I should not bother to stop at the gym? Should I get a standing desk?

No, I am not telling you to skip the gym, and no, you don't necessarily have to get a standing desk. While they do offer benefits, they cost money, and standing all day has negative health consequences, too.

A good solution, according to Dr. James Levine, is to get up for ten minutes every hour, and walk around a bit rather than just standing. Dr. Joan Vernikos, former NASA Life Sciences director

---

51 Soritsa, D., "Maternal physical activity and sedentary behaviour before and during in vitro fertilization treatment: a longitudinal study exploring the associations with controlled ovarian stimulation and pregnancy outcomes," *J Assist Reprod Genet.* 2020 Aug;37(8):1869-1881

and author of *Sitting Kills, Moving Heals*, believes that getting up from sitting 35 times per day is what's needed.[52]

I don't know if "sitting kills," but it does contribute to back pain. While I am always happy to treat back pain in my fertility patients, too many of you are suffering from it at a young age.

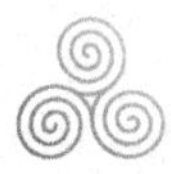

52 Vernikos, J., *Sitting Kills, Moving Heals: How Everyday Movement Will Prevent Pain, Illness, and Early Dath—and Exercise Alone Won't*, Quill Driver Books, 2011

Exercise snacks

I read somewhere that just short bursts of intense exercise can be helpful. Should I do that when I take my stand-up breaks?

GREAT IDEA. IN ONE STUDY, even an 11-minute burst was beneficial. But there are important details here.

"Exercise snacks" is a term coined by exercise physiologist Monique Francois to describe short bursts of exercise that seemed to show beneficial effects. The idea to look at this grew out of a mortality study of 50,000 people who mostly sat all day. It showed that people who moved—even a little bit, for 10 or 11 minutes—lived longer than people who moved about for only two to three minutes per day.

Although longevity is important to you, it is different from your more immediate goals of increasing energy and losing weight. More vigorous activity (as opposed to just getting up out of one's chair in the previous study) for short amounts does have benefits. Research at McMaster University showed that people who raced up three flights of stairs, three times per day, for three days per week, showed improved leg strength and aerobic capacity. This 20-second "exercise snack" fits the definition of vigorous activity. Vigorous bursts of activity for fitness were also popularized several years ago by Chris Jordan, an exercise physiologist at the Johnson and Johnson Human Performance Institute. His "seven-minute workout" requires just a floor, chairs, and a wall, but it is extremely intense and could lead to injuries if a person is not quite up to it. Consider looking at the readily available videos, and then create your own version of a seven-minute workout, tailoring it to your needs.

While just getting up from the computer at intervals and short bursts of exercise can be beneficial, consistent and moderately vigorous consistent walking is often and ultimately the best way to go.

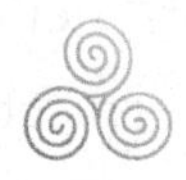

Refreshing You and Your Home

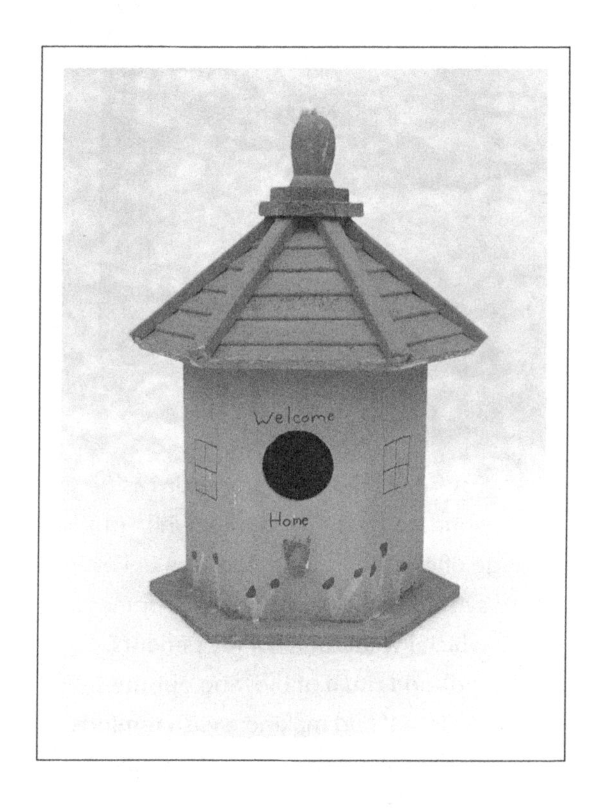

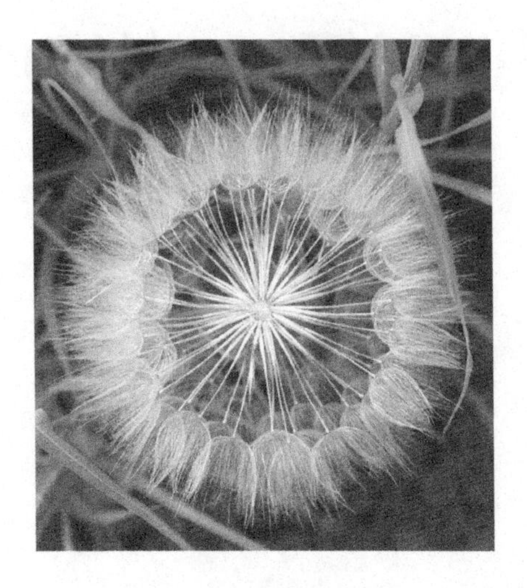

Potential medicinal properties aside, dandelions are beautiful in their white puffball stage of exposed seeds. They are believed to symbolize hope, love, and happiness which I want for all of my patients. The childhood ritual of blowing out the seeds to fertile soil and making a wish reminds me of the pop psychology strategy of putting wishes out to the Universe to attract what you desire.

A conversation over tea

Dandelions are in the asteraceae family of flowers along with daises, sunflowers, and chamomile plants. The roots, stems, and leaves can be used to make tea. It has been used in traditional medicine to treat liver problems and as a diuretic.

I invite you to try some dandelion tea for its theoretical ability to assist the liver. The liver and kidneys do the big job of filtering chemicals, hormones, and waste products from the blood. These waste products leave the liver through its production of bile, and the kidney through its urine. Dandelions are high in bioactive substances called polysaccharides, which the liver needs to make bile. So perhaps this could be how dandelions enhance liver function. Dandelion tea is safe but may interact with certain antibiotics like ciprofloxacin and levofloxacin. If you are allergic to ragweed, daises, marigolds, and chrysanthemums, there might be some cross-allergy with dandelions.[53]

---

53 Wirngo, FE, "The Physiological Effects of Dandelion (*Taraxacum Officinale*) in Type 2 Diabetes," *Rev Diabet Stud. 2016 Summer-Fall; 13(2-3): 113–131*

An ounce of prevention

THE LIVER AND KIDNEYS CANNOT REMOVE all toxins from your body, in part because some of the toxins migrate to body fat, where they remain. The key to keeping toxins and toxics out of your body is to avoid exposure and intake in the first place.

To clarify, "toxins" refers to harmful substances in nature, such as poison mushrooms, snake venom, arsenic, or lead. "Toxics" refers to man-made chemicals that are harmful, like pesticides and industrial-waste products that seep into rivers, oceans, groundwater, air, and some of the foods we eat. I want to make sure you know some things about both.

My intent is to empower you to protect your health by adding to your body of knowledge on harmful substances and how to avoid them. This part of our conversation may cause some distress, but I promise a "good news" and positive ending to this section.

We are at war—a biochemical war—and the enemy is lurking in our environment. We eat, drink, absorb, and breathe harmful substances every day. Not even newborn babies are safe and often are born with more than 200 environmental chemicals in their blood from maternal exposure.[54] In the last 60 years, increased rates of obesity, hormone-dependent cancers, chronic childhood disease, developmental disorders, poor birth outcomes, and longer time to pregnancy "are unlikely to be explained solely by genetic mutations, therefore warranting consideration of other causes, including the environment."[55]

Hormone-disrupting chemicals used to harden or soften plastic leach out of containers and products and have negative effects on hormones. Pesticides and herbicides cause cancer and birth defects, and hang out in the food chain forever. Water can be unsafe, depending on the source and its level of bacteria, metals, and chemicals. The government is trying its best to protect us while balancing the needs of industry, but troubling challenges remain. You can and need to act to protect yourself.

Obviously, cute, smart, and wonderful babies are conceived and born every day despite the toxics in us. But our species may be reaching a breaking point, and we do not know enough about the potential health hazards. "Although the field of reproductive environmental health is still in its infancy, the stakes are high."[56]

After going through IVF cycles, giving birth, or having a miscarriage, you may want to re-establish regular periods and optimal

54 Miller, M, "Toxic Exposure: Chemicals Are in Our Water, Food, Air and Furniture: Are the Chemicals We Encounter Every Day Making Us Sick?" https://www.ucsf.edu/news/2017/06/407416/toxic-exposure-chemicals-are-in-our-water-food-air-and-furniture?utm_source=email&utm_medium=edu&utm_campaign=environmental%20toxics

55 Smarr, M, "Endocrine-Distrupting Chemicals and Endometriosis," *Fertility and Sterility*, Vol. 106 September 15, 2016

56 *Ibid.*

hormonal functioning while deciding what your next steps will be. After reproductive challenges, many of my patients tell me they just want to get back to feeling energetic, interested in sex, and hopeful about the future. Whether your goal is to have optimal hormonal function, healthier eggs, healthier sperm, less risk of cancer, or more longevity, reducing the number of environmental chemicals in your body is a good strategy.

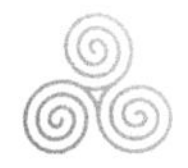

Who stole your sperm?

I THOUGHT ABOUT MAKING THIS THE SUBTITLE to this book of our conversations. There is ample evidence that men's fertility is impacted by endocrine-disrupting toxics.[57,58]

Sperm quality and quantity is an issue for about one third of couples struggling to conceive. Sperm counts have gone down steadily each decade, with a 59% drop between 1973 and 2011.[59] The quality of sperm has decreased as well, as evidenced by an increase in abnormal shapes, including missing heads, two heads, missing tails, and inability to swim well.

Women often feel responsible for miscarrying their baby, but the fact is that many miscarriages are due to genetic reasons, and

---

57 Rehman, S., "Endocrine-disrupting chemicals and impact on male reproductive health," *Transl Androl Urol.* 2018 Jun; 7(3): 490–503

58 *Ibid.*

59 Swan, S, *Countdown: How Our Modern World Is Threatening Sperm Counts, Altering Male and Female Reproductive Development, and Imperiling the Future of the Human Race*, Scribner 2020, Page 50

from the moment of conception, half the genes are from the man, and half from the woman. As sperm quality has gone down, the risk of miscarriages has gone up. Professor of Environmental Medicine Shanna Swan writes that, "Between 2002 and 2012, the incidence of recurrent miscarriages increased by 74% among a cohort of 6,852 Swedish women ages 18 to 42. That's a rapid increase in the span of just nine years.[60] Some of Dr. Swan's conclusions have been challenged. One reason for this, according to Dr. Allen Pacey, andrologist and editor of *Human Fertility*, "sperm counting is tricky business and notoriously prone to error."[61] Nonetheless, sorting out the reasons for and treating declining sperm counts are not a huge priority for Western medicine. After all, there are plenty of people on the planet, and the availability of the IVF recipe of one sperm per egg plus one cup of hormones removes a sense of urgency.

But men have a lot more on the line besides low sperm count, which is often just a sign of the damage being done by toxics to thyroid function and testosterone production, which lead to weight gain, fatigue, low libido, and erectile dysfunction. These health problems start with hormone disruption, but men are also vulnerable to higher rates of cancers associated with certain pollutants.

I bought something called De-tox tea. Will it help me be less toxic?
First of all, *you* are not toxic—the environment is. Unfortunately, for many years we have absorbed toxics from air, water, food, and products.

"De-tox" teas, which are usually blends of herbal teas like dandelion and nettle leaf, cannot remove all the hormone-disrupting

60 *Ibid*.

61 Gross, RE, "The Sperm Count 'Crisis' Doesn't Add Up," *The New York Times*, June 4, 2020

and cancer-causing chemicals we harbor. Some herbs will have a diuretic effect on the body, and some will stimulate your bowels to move, but that does not mean that all of the dangerous environmental chemicals leave your body with your waste products.

There is no evidence that juice diets and colonic irrigation (enemas) can eliminate harmful chemicals, either. I worry about my patients who regularly see a "colonic hydro therapist" for enemas, because bowel perforation and electrolyte imbalance can occur with enemas. It's not wise to take this risk when there is no research to prove its effectiveness. The natural bacteria in the colon break down toxics and move them out through stool. Mucous membranes in the gut keep toxics from being reabsorbed.

I use only plastic things labeled "BPA-free," so I am safe from toxics in plastic, right?

Not completely, but I am glad you asked this question.

"BPA" short for *bisphenol A*, is in a group of chemicals called *endocrine disruptors* because they disrupt the function of our endocrine glands, including the thyroid, ovaries, testes, pancreas, and adrenal glands. These glands produce important hormones such as estrogen, progesterone, testosterone, thyroxin, insulin, and cortisol. These hormones were never meant to compete with the likes of BPA.

It is not surprising that BPA disrupts estrogen, as it was originally manufactured back in the 1930s as a synthetic estrogen for women suffering from miscarriages. That use was abandoned early on, but somebody in a lab realized BPA was a great agent for hardening plastics. Now more than nine million pounds of BPA are produced annually for food and beverage containers.

The problem is that plastic is an unstable compound and breaks down when it gets too old, too warm, or too cold and releases BPA into the contents of the container, which we then consume. Our bodies are understandably confused and thrown off balance when BPA enters, as its chemical configuration looks like estrogen. In addition to reproductive-hormone disruption, BPA and its chemical cousins are suspected "obesogens" and "diabetogens," because they might be slowing down the thyroid gland, leading to insulin resistance and weight gain, which, in turn, is associated with Type 2 diabetes.

In an effort to address consumer alarm and decrease the disruptive effects of BPA, the plastics industry tweaked the formula and renamed it "BPAS," "BPAF," and "BPAB." Some scientists believe that these new chemical cousins are even more disruptive than BPA.[62]

The bottom line is that a product can be labeled "BPA-free" and still cause hormonal disruption.

In addition to BPA, there are other chemicals you want to avoid to enhance hormonal balance. Phthalate, which is a great Scrabble word but a harmful chemical, is used as a plastic softener in hundreds of products such as medical tubing, blood containers, food-storage containers, adhesives, toys, soap, shampoo, nail polish, and lotions. Most exposure comes from eating and drinking foods that have been in containers containing phthalates. A growing body of evidence shows that phthalates

62 Eladak, S., "A new chapter in the bisphenol A story: bisphenol S and bisphenol F are not safe alternatives to this compound," *Fertility and Sterility.* 2015 Jan;103(1):11-21.

negatively affect sperm and may have a role in development of uterine fibroids.[63]

Other chemicals added to many lotions and potions include parabens and tricolosan. Parabens are synthetic chemicals used as a preservative for soaps, cosmetics, and personal-care products, so their main route of entry is through the skin. Like BPA, all of the paraben cousins are considered endocrine disruptors and *xenoestrogens*. Xeno (pronounced *zeno*) comes from the Greek root for "strange" or "foreign." These chemicals do, indeed, look to the body like estrogen, but a strange or foreign one that interferes with endocrine function. The Environmental Working Group (EWG.org) has a list of current research on the disruptive effects of parabens.[64] Like other endocrine disruptors, parabens have a short half-life, meaning that they are metabolized and eliminated by the body quickly, but some is left behind in tissues. The good news is that there are plenty of paraben-free personal-care products.

Scan labels for ingredients like methylparaben, ethylparaben, propylparaben, and butylparaben. Multiple abbreviations for each are used on labels. For example, methylparaben can be listed as "MP," "MeP," "MPB," "MePB," or "MePben." Don't worry about memorizing these letters—I will be giving you some ways to find paraben-free products.

Triclosan is a synthetic antibacterial chemical used in laundry detergent, dish soap, hand soap, and toothpaste. It is even added to some textiles to make them more resistant to bacteria. Scientists

---

63 Zota, A., "Phthalates exposure and uterine-fibroid burden among women undergoing surgical treatment for fibroids: a preliminary study," *Fertility and Sterility*, January 1, 2019, 112-121

64 Stoiber, T., "What Are Parabens, and Why Don't They Belong in Cosmetics?" April, 9, 2019, https://www.ewg.org/californiacosmetics/parabens)

believe we probably don't get much antibacterial protection from it; so, there is no reason to expose yourself to its cancer-causing and endocrine-disrupting potential. Although triclosan is found in the urine of 75% of the people tested, we have only a few human studies that show a direct link to endocrine disruption. But the chickens, rats, and monkeys that were studied had huge problems with their placentas and estradiol levels when exposed to triclosan. My fertility patient Amanda is a physical therapist in a nursing home. She washed her hands before and after each patient about 15 times per day. I suggested she check the label on the soap provided at the facility. She was very unhappy and frustrated when she saw that it listed triclosan. I suggested an easy solution: bring your own soap to work. Again, it is the frequent and cumulative exposure that is a problem, not occasional use of a product.

Nothing lasts forever . . . except certain chemicals

PERSISTENT ORGANIC POLLUTANTS (POPS) are another category of chemicals that you should avoid. They are referred to as "forever chemicals," because it takes a very long time for them to be excreted from the body, and they never leave the environment. If you had a measurable blood level of one type of "forever chemical" called a PFAS (polyfluoroalkyl substance) but were never exposed again, you would still have half of that level in four years. With chemical abbreviations like PFOA, PFOs, PBDE, PCDE, and PFAs, they are used in coatings for products to make them more resistant to oil, grease, or water. Consequently, they are found in food packaging, non-stick coatings, textiles, and paper, as well as herbicides and pesticides. They enter us when we drink water contaminated by industrial runoff and eat foods from coated packaging. Hand to mouth, as in eating finger foods after touching waterproof fabrics or carpets, is another mode of transmission. Research has linked these chemicals to immune, endocrine, developmental, and neurologic disease. Although some have been banned, like PCB in 1979, they live on in our oceans and soil, which results in exposure through eating fish and plants. Although we can try to avoid coated products, the cows, chickens, and pigs that we eat have eaten plants and grains from soil contaminated with pesticides and herbicides and pass it on to us. Fish swimming in water contaminated from agricultural runoff are another source.

Exactly what levels of these various "forever chemicals" cause cancer, reproductive, immune, and neurological problems is difficult for scientists to determine. Chemical manufacturers and consumer-protection groups cannot seem to agree on what blood and tissue level is safe or what amount of exposure will lead to those levels. We do know that agricultural workers have disproportionately higher rates of "birth defects, neurological complications, respiratory illness, and cancers."[65]

It is very good news that levels of certain "forever chemicals" (PFAs) have started to decline, according to David Andrews, PhD, toxicologist and Senior analyst at the Environmental Working Group, a non-profit consumer-advocacy organization. "On the positive side, we have seen a decrease in the last decade of concentration of PFAs in our blood, based on a voluntary phase-out agreement that the manufacturers entered into with the EPA. We have seen that changes in the chemical marketplace do lead to changes in the general population and how much they're exposed.

65 "Dangerous Exposure: Farmworker Children and Pesticides," published in the *The Fields Health and Safety Programs Annual Publication*, 2011. https://afop.org/wp-content/uploads/2010/07/Annual_Publication_FINAL_English1.pdf

We've also learned more about how potent these chemicals are and how much more needs to be done. "But change absolutely can happen, and it can happen in our lifetime."[66]

Change did happen recently in Minnesota, according to a recent study published in the *Environmental Health Journal.* It showed that "The rate of premature births and low-weight births in Oakdale, Minnesota, dropped dramatically, and fertility rates increased after the city began filtering PFAs from its tap water."[67]

Are non-organic fruits and vegetables really a significant source of toxics that may be harmful?

With one billion pounds of pesticides used per year, mostly on crops, this information is not surprising. Even if a certain level is determined to be safe, it seems reasonable that individual responses, just like individual responses to alcohol or allergens, could be a factor that would be difficult to determine.

I try to keep up with peer-reviewed research in medical journals, but the study that got my attention on eating organic was done in 2013 by middle-school student Ria Chhabra for her science project. She boxed up two groups of fruit flies and fed organic produce to one and non-organic to the other. The fruit flies who feasted on organic fruits and vegetables produced many more offspring and lived longer than the flies who were fed non-organic produce. Female fruit flies lay hundreds of eggs (as all of us who keep bananas too long know), and their life span is about eight

---

66 https://www.huffpost.com/entry/forever-chemicals-food-pfas_l_5cfa7d79e4b0c7edd0b6591e)

67 "Minn. Study Is First to Show Cause-and-Effect Link Between 'Forever Chemicals' in Drinking Water and Reproductive Harms," https://www.ewg.org/news-and-analysis/2020/09/minn-study-first-show-cause-and-effect-link-between-forever-chemicals

to ten days. Ria must have spent a lot of time counting the little pests. Her results caught the attention of academic researchers, who repeated her methodology in a university fly lab. It showed similar results. This inspired human studies in which the data strongly supports the positive benefits of eating organic.[68,69]

Consumer demand for organic produce has increased competition and lowered prices. Frozen organic foods are sometimes less expensive, and, in general, the nutrients are preserved. If organic food is not within your budget or available, wash fruits and vegetables for at least 20 seconds under cold running water, followed by brushing or wiping them. This does not remove all bad chemicals, because some seep through the peels and wax coatings trap them inside, but it will remove most.

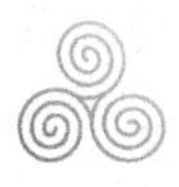

68 Vigar, V., "A Systematic Review of Organic Versus Conventional Food Consumption: Is There a Measurable Benefit on Human Health?" *Nutrients*. 2020 Jan; 12(1): 7

69 https://www.ncbi.nlm.nih.gov/pmc/articles/PMC7019963/

Water, water, everywhere

BUT NOT A DROP TO DRINK. This line is from the 1798 poem *The Rime of the Ancient Mariner* by Samuel Coleridge and was attributed to a sailor stranded on a becalmed (and salty) sea, dying of thirst. It seems as if we are surrounded by water options, but much of it contains stuff I would rather you not drink when trying to Refresh.

I drink only bottled water, so I am safe, right?

Not necessarily. Chemicals leach out of plastic, and unless you routinely drink the expensive Italian and French water in glass bottles, you may be needlessly exposing yourself to hormone disruptors.

Bottled water comes in a dizzying array of options and is labeled as:

* "Purified," which usually means that it came out of the tap and has some, but not all, chemicals filtered out.

* "Spring," from underground and may or may not be purified.

* "Mineral," from springs that contain carbon dioxide making it "bubbly"

* "Sparkling," usually from the tap with carbon dioxide pumped into it to make it bubbly. Think seltzer water.

But all this water, whether from the tap or in a bottle, comes to us from lakes, rivers, and underground springs. This sounds pristine but unfortunately contains:

* Waterborne pathogens (bacteria) from birds and animals

* Runoff water from farms containing pesticides and herbicides

* Industrial chemicals dumped into waterways

* Natural toxins (like arsenic) from soil that seeps into springs

* Lead or bacteria from pipes used for transport

* Endocrine-disrupting chemicals from plastic containers.

* Hormones, because people pee them out or flush them down the toilet

These potential exposures can negatively impact health and healing. The Environmental Protection Agency, our government agency in charge of monitoring and reporting water issues, has written that, "If drinking water contains unsafe levels of contaminants, it can cause health effects such as gastrointestinal illnesses, nervous system or reproductive effects, and chronic diseases such as cancer . . ."[70]

There is ongoing debate and non-consensus between health scientists and industry scientists about the levels of contaminants in water that are deemed unsafe. But there is no debate that much of the water we drink contains things from the list I mentioned.

Should I just try to wean myself off bottled water and filter my water on my own? What kind of filter is best?

I have researched water filters and would love to give you a definitive answer. But there are so many on the market, all claiming to be the best. Part of the challenge is that there is no one filter or process that can remove all types of contaminants. For example, carbon filters remove chlorine, sediment, odor, and taste. Reverse-osmosis filters remove heavy metals and microbes. A combination of the two types may reduce but not completely eliminate hormones found in water. I did view one expensive filtration product whose manufacturer claimed that its filter removed 99.9% of every known contaminant. But the only research done was by the manufacturer and was not independently verified.

I am handing the research over to you. Please tell me what you find. I know I keep mentioning the Environmental Working Group.org, but that is because they are a great independent source for information on things like water filters.

---

70 https://www.epa.gov/ground-water-and-drinking-water

Bottled water is sometimes unavoidable when we travel or are on the run. Don't worry about that. Our amazing bodies can handle some contaminants. Some bottled-water companies do filter their water, but the efficacy of their processes is not routinely monitored by outside agencies. And the bigger problem remains—that even if environmental contaminants are removed by filtration, plastic chemicals from the bottle may continue to infuse the water. Not drinking from bottles exposed to extreme temperatures and a long time on a shelf can reduce your risk.

You can keep things simple for yourself by drinking home-filtered tap water in glass or stainless steel containers. It's best to have your water checked for lead, copper, and other metals if you are unsure about your pipes. If you have a well, have it checked once a year for bacteria. Municipalities and private companies offer test kits. If you are concerned about bacteria or don't like the taste and smell of your tap water, try boiling a few day's worth of drinking water at a time, and storing it in glass or stainless-steel containers. If you choose to use a carbon-filter system that empties into a plastic pitcher (as most of them do), transfer the water after filtering to glass or stainless steel for storage and drinking.

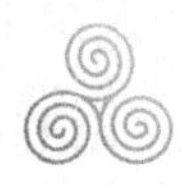

Mother Nature could not have known

WHILE ON THE TOPIC of potentially harmful substances, we need to talk about the "natural ones." Even substances that come from the plants, animals, and minerals around us are not necessarily safe. Think poison ivy and arsenic. Remember the chart you had to memorize in school called the "Periodic Table"? It is a list of the natural substances that have lived in the Earth's crust since our planet was formed 4.5 billion years ago. There are 118 substances or elements. Names that may ring a bell are lead, cadmium, zinc, and aluminum. The combination of these elements forms the sturdy, round ball we call planet Earth. Small amounts of some elements meet important nutritional needs, and we get them by eating the plants that have soaked them up from the ground.

Mother Nature could not have known that we would slather on zinc sunscreens and aluminum antiperspirants. I worry when a patient tells me that they are supplementing their prenatal vitamins with high doses of zinc because they heard it was good for fertility.

High levels of zinc can cause GI disturbances as well as impair immunity, even though, in small amounts, it can help immunity. One study revealed that teen girls who apply cadmium-laden lipstick and gloss as much as 20 times per day had alarmingly high blood levels to show for it. Cadmium, used for everything from batteries to cosmetics, probably does not pass through the skin but is ingested by the mouth's mucous membranes when lipstick is applied. High levels of cadmium can cause kidney and liver damage and may be carcinogenic at high doses. There is not much consensus among scientists on what dose or blood level of the "heavy metal" elements can cause health problems, but it is best not to be complacent about products and to keep checking back with scientists.

How am I supposed to remember which are the safe products?
Don't worry. There is, as they say, "an app for that." As well as plenty of databases and some very good non-profits trying to educate us.

Some good sources of information about which cosmetics are safer than others can be found on the EWG.org site and at FDA Consumer Updates, https://www.fda.gov/cosmetics/cosmetics-labeling-regulations/cosmetics-labeling-guide. Some of my patients use the "Think Dirty "app, which allows you to scan barcodes to get information on whether the product may contain harmful substances. The Silent Spring Institute, whose mission involves the environment and women's health, has a great "DetoxMe" app (https://wwww.silentspring.org/detoxmeactionkit/) that can point you in the right direction.

The most efficient way to an ounce of prevention is to put in the time to find safe products you like and then stick with them, rather than use apps while shopping or scour databases on a regular basis.

What's the deal with GMOs?

I cannot answer that, but I don't feel dumb. Even scientists who have been studying this topic cannot agree on whether genetically modified organisms (GMOs) pose a health risk.

Genetically modified organisms (GMOs) are plants whose genes have been altered to make them sweeter (think corn) or more resistant to weed killers. It is this latter quality that alarms environmentalists who believe that toxic weed killers are used more liberally because a plant's altered genes keep it safe from destruction by the weed killer. The GMO industry and the pesticide makers deny that creating pesticide- and herbicide-resistant plants has led to increased use of weed killers. A pro-GMO website states that the creation of weed- and bug-killer-resistant plants has led to a slight (8%) decrease in pesticide use. Regardless of what the deal is, we should all at least support efforts to require that GMO foods are labeled, so we can choose for ourselves whether to eat them.

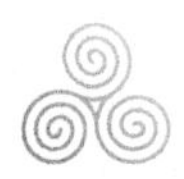

Chemicals in the drugs you need and maybe don't need

I have been taking anti-depressants since freshman year in college. I have a prescription for an anti-anxiety med if I need it. Should I stop taking them?

IF YOU WILL BE TRYING TO CONCEIVE AGAIN after you Renourish and Revitalize, there are some things to consider.

One, whether anti-depressants decrease fertility, and two, whether it is safe for your baby to be exposed to them *in utero*. There are negative and positive studies in the medical literature in regard to anti-depressants and women's fertility. A recent meta-analysis concludes "There is insufficient evidence at present to propose that SSRIs reduce fertility or fertility-treatment outcome."[71]

---

71 Sylvester, C., "Selective Serotonin Reuptake Inhibitors and Fertility: Considerations for Couples Trying to Conceive," *Harvard Review of Psychiatry*. Mar/Apr 2019;27(2):108-118

The research on men and SSRIs is more clear and shows an association between SSRI use and sperm parameters.[72]

Sperm is obviously easier to study than women's eggs because samples can simply be obtained easily pre- and post-SSRI use. Fortunately, the research seems to indicate that the effects of SSRIs are reversible when treatment is discontinued.

An association between anti-depressants and first-trimester pregnancy loss has been observed, but it may depend on the type of anti-depressant used. More research is needed on this and the question of whether underlying depression and not anti-depressants have caused reproductive problems for some people.

Getting back to your question about whether you should try to go off of your anti-depressants: I can tell you that most of my patients' doctors are supportive of women continuing anti-depressive therapy in their reproductive years, given the dangers of major depression. However, most of my patients express some degree of concern and guilt about taking them. If you have mild to moderate depression and want to wean off anti-depressants, plan to do it very slowly under the direction of the prescribing doctor. Withdrawal schedules are based on type, dose, and length of time you have been on the medication, but no less than 6 weeks (and potentially much longer) may be suggested by many practitioners to avoid a rebound of the depression. "If women are trying to avoid possible risk to a baby, and their depression has been tolerable and without suicide concerns, they could go off moderate doses of anti-depressants in several weeks, as long as

---

72 Beeder, L., "Effect of antidepressant medications on semen parameters and male fertility," *J Urol.* 2020 Jan;27(1):39-46

they understand they might have discontinuation symptoms."[73] "Discontinuation symptoms" can include flu-like symptoms, nausea, vertigo, sleep disturbances, agitations, anxiety, and sensory disturbances like electric-shock sensations. According to psychiatrist Dr. Kenneth Robbins, these symptoms can last as long as a month, but rarely longer.

If you decide to discontinue anti-depressants, have a plan to exercise more, meditate more, eat well, and sleep well. These things and complementary methods such as acupuncture have all been shown to help lessen depression.

In addition to anti-depressants, there are other prescription medications that may affect a man's sperm. This includes anti-hypertensives (calcium channel blockers), anti-inflammatories (sulfasalazine for inflammatory bowel disease), acid reducers for heartburn and GERD (cimetidine), and hair loss preparations like finasteride (trade name Propecia.) In each category of these medications, there are kinder alternatives for sperm that your doctor can help you figure out. For some conditions like mild hypertension and heartburn, diet and exercise can eliminate the need for prescription medications, but do not discontinue a prescribed medication without advice and guidance from your doctor.

My husband likes to smoke marijuana. He should probably quit if we decide to keep trying to conceive, right?

---

73 Conversation with Dr. Kenneth Robbins, Psychiatrist and Adjunct Professor, University of Wisconsin, May 2021

Right. If you will be trying to conceive in the future, know that the THC in marijuana can decrease sperm count, motility, and libido.[74]

A 2015 study done in Denmark showed that sperm counts were 29% lower in men who smoked marijuana once per week, and the more they smoked, the lower they went.[75]

Studies are less clear about the association of ovum quality and marijuana, but research with animals indicates the two important hormones, luteinizing hormone and follicle-stimulating hormone, were affected by THC, the active ingredient in marijuana.[76]

In addition to this, women undergoing fertility treatment who smoked marijuana "had more than double the miscarriage rate of those who didn't."[77]

If your goal is to maintain or enhance fertility while deciding on your next steps, choosing not to smoke or eat marijuana could be a good decision. If you use marijuana for relaxation, also note that chronic heavy use is associated with depression.

CBD oil is from marijuana, but it's safe, right?

I can't say for sure, but CBD is a derivative of cannabis and may have some of its negative reproductive effects.

There are small amounts of CBD (cannabidiol) oil in marijuana plants, but much of our supply of CBD oil comes from the hemp plant, which is a botanical cousin of the marijuana. Both hemp and marijuana are in a plant family known as *cannabis sativa.*

---

74 Hsiao, P., "Adverse Effects of Cannabis on Male Reproduction," https://www.ncbi.nlm.nih.gov/pubmed/30146239 *Eur Urol Focus.* 2018 Apr;4(3):324-328

75 Swan, S., *Count Down.* 2020 Page 96.

76 Smith, CG, "Acute, short-term, and chronic effects of marijuana on the female primate reproductive function," *A Res Monogr.* 1984;44:82-96.

77 Swan, *op. cit.*, p. 96

CBD has very little of the psychoactive THC found in marijuana and has been approved for use as an anti-epileptic. Its use for inflammation, anxiety, and pain is being studied. Some patients have told me CBD oil helps them sleep, while others have said they feel no effect at all. While some dispensaries are touting CBD as a fertility enhancer, there is inadequate data to support these claims. Animal studies have shown that CBD decreased testicular size and reduced the ability of sperm to fertilize eggs.[78] As with many supplements, CBD products are not always labeled correctly in terms of strength or purity, which may cause some of the problems with it. A study in the *Journal of the American Medical Association* found problems with 43% of online products.[79]

My brother smokes pot, and my sister-in-law microwaves in plastic. They have four kids. How do you explain that?
Easily. And *not* with the answer used by industries—that your relative's fertility proves chemicals are not harmful.

When covered in yellow pollen each spring after cleaning my screened porch, I never sneeze, not even once. I think I could jump into a vat of pollen and be fine. Some patients come into my office and sneeze if I have fresh flowers, or even plastic ones with dust on them. If I drink two beers, I need a nap; my husband is safe to drive after two beers. Just like with allergies, substances affect people differently depending on their "constitution" and genetic makeup. Your brother, sister-in-law, and other people may

---

78 Evans, D., "Medical Fraud, Mislabeling, Contamination: All Common in CBD Products," *Mo Med.* 2020 Sept-Oct; 117:394-399

79 Bonn-Miller, M., "Labeling Accuracy of Cannabidiol Extracts Sold online." *JAMA* 2017 Nov. 7 318(17): 1708-1709

be less sensitive to endocrine disruption by chemicals. I call this the Jane Gleeson Theory of Relativity: An individual's blood levels of disruptors can be measured, but, unfortunately, we don't have a good blood test for sensitivity to those chemicals. An ounce of prevention would still be the main solution.

I'm sorry, but all this information about chemicals and toxins has just added to my anxiety. I can't really control all this exposure anyway, right?
I am the one who needs to apologize for making you feel anxious. The thought of what we are exposed to is overwhelming, and you are correct: we cannot control a lot of it.

We would probably have to live in a bubble to get away from all plastics, and the bubble would probably have to be made of plastic or some bad chemical. Similarly, you cannot walk around with a respirator to clean the air you breathe. But you can control your exposure by making some simple choices and forming some easy habits, and it will be worth your while. There was a very interesting study done by a woman obstetrician in which a small group of families was sequestered and provided with food that had never touched plastic. In two weeks, the subject's urine BPA levels had dropped 66%.[80]

The kidneys try to clear BPA, which is why checking urine is an easy way to measure levels. But some always stays in the body and is stored in fat. It would probably be impossible to have zero BPA and other chemicals in our systems, given our chronic

80 Rudel, R., "Food Packaging and Bisphenol A and Bis(2-Ethyhexyl) Phthalate Exposure: Findings from a Dietary Intervention," open access https://ehp.niehs.nih.gov/doi/10.1289/ehp.1003170?url_ver=Z39.88-200pubmed

exposure, but zero need not be the goal. Just getting the levels lower can, hopefully, reduce disruption and enhance health.

Read labels for chemicals you want to avoid, pick your products, stick with them, and you won't have to keep checking everything. I have made these lists to help you simplify your approach and lessen anxiety about contaminants.

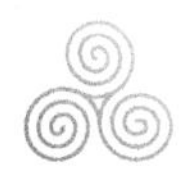

Simple checklists for clean eating and clean nesting

EAT FRESH OR FROZEN FRUITS AND VEGETABLES instead of canned ones. BPA and BPA-type products are often used to line cans.

Eat organic when possible. I know you commented about the price, but when you pay a bit more for that peach, you will be more likely to eat it rather than let it spoil while you grab some chips.

Choose lean meats, because many toxic substances build up in animal fat. That is where they are stored in us as well. Trim the fat off meat and the skin off of fish before cooking.

Cook in stainless steel, glass, cast iron, or enameled cast iron pans. Get rid of your non-stick coated pans. Even the manufacturers of some non-stick coatings admit that chemicals leach out at 500 degrees.

Store leftovers in glass or stainless-steel containers. Glass bowls are fine, even if they have plastic lids—just don't lick the applesauce off the lids.

Drink from glass or stainless steel containers. Remember, "BPA Free" is not necessarily safe, as the chemical that has replaced it has recently been found to be an endocrine disruptor. If you drink bottled water, do not let it bake or freeze in your car, and don't refill bottles.

Buy as many staples as possible in glass. Peanut butter, jams, pickles, mayonnaise, ketchup, and mustard all come in glass. You may have to look for them and pay a bit more, but this is a small price to pay and a source of exposure that you can control. The jars are great for snacks and leftovers—it really saves on wax-paper and aluminum foil use.

Use caution when handling thermal paper of the type used for many credit-card receipts and ATMs. It is coated with BPA so that the ink won't smear. It doesn't necessarily go through your skin but can be ingested if you pick up food without washing your hands.

Clean household interiors and washable items with baking soda, vinegar, or castile soap, which is made from vegetable oil. You can buy huge bags of baking soda and gallons of vinegar at a fraction of the cost of "Bubbly Foaming" cleanser in a plastic bottle.

Hand wash plastic dishes and utensils. Hot dishwashers may melt the plastic of the dishes, washing the those chemicals onto your glass dishes and metal utensils.

Have a shoeless house. Shoes can carry toxic chemicals into your home. Some guests may think it is weird when you ask them to remove their shoes, but just tell them you were Japanese in your other life. I keep socks and shoe covers at my door, and always advise dinner guests that they may want to wear socks without holes. You will notice that your carpeting and wood floors will look and feel cleaner for longer periods of time when you leave shoes at the door.

Choose upholstered furniture and rugs made from wool or cotton fibers that have not been treated with flame retardants and stain-resistant chemicals.

Damp-mop your floors rather than sweep them, because lead, pesticides, and flame retardants are swept into the air you breathe as you sweep. Lead and pesticides come in with your dog or cat, since they probably don't wear shoes that you can take off. Mopping often or wiping animal feet may be a solution.

Hand wash delicate clothing and sweaters to reduce exposure to dry-cleaning chemicals. If necessary, choose a dry cleaner who uses the "wet" process rather than using PERC (perchloroethylene) to clean. Clothes made from natural and organic fibers are comfortable and easy to wash, but a few chemically laden, no-iron or stain-resistant items in your closet are okay.

Be kind to bugs and yourself by not using too many pesticides for non-threatening insects like ants and some (I emphasize *some*) spiders. Of course, we need to protect ourselves from bedbugs, ticks, and mosquitoes. There are many recipes on the Internet for repellents that are composed of vinegar and essential oils from eucalyptus and lemon. These less toxic alternatives have been shown to work.

Please don't stress about contaminants, toxics, and toxins. If you are planning to conceive, remember: beautiful, smart, healthy babies are conceived and born every day. But when you are trying to do everything that you can to be healthy, heal, or enhance fertility, it is important to be armed with information.

If you are interested in what you can do on a bigger scale, pay attention to what you read or hear about laws being considered in your state or on the federal level that will protect you from chemical, air, and water pollution. I guarantee that, if you read news in your state, you will see articles almost every day about consumer-protection bills that never make it out of committee due to the lobbying efforts of big business. I like the response of Dr. Chan (Harvard Exposure Assessment scientist) on the pushback from industry regarding chemicals: "'Innocent until proven guilty' may be the right starting point for criminal justice, but it is disastrous chemical policy."[81] Write, e-mail, or call your congressional representatives to express your concerns. Industries have professional lobbyists who work full time, but collectively we have a loud voice.

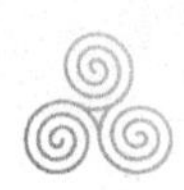

81 Swan, S., Opinion piece in *The Washington Post* quoted in *Count Down*, 2016

Rebalancing and Next Steps

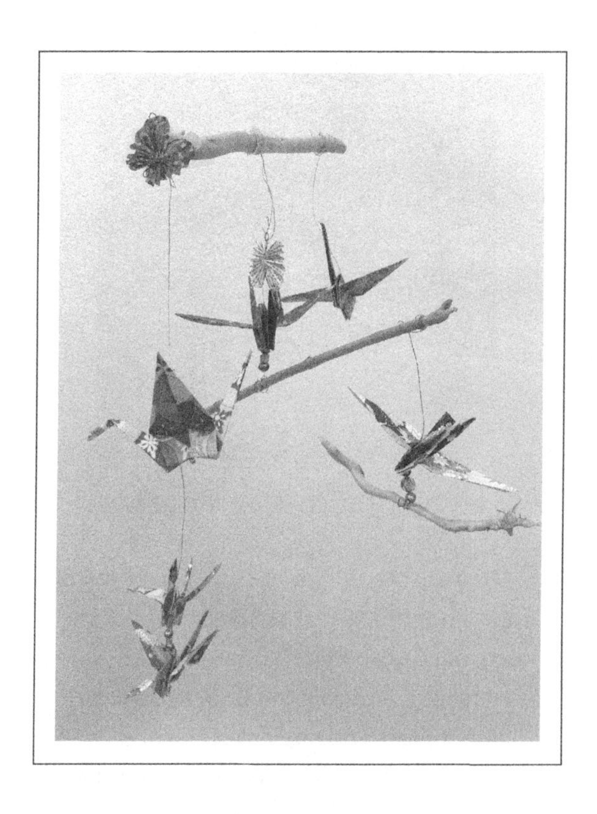

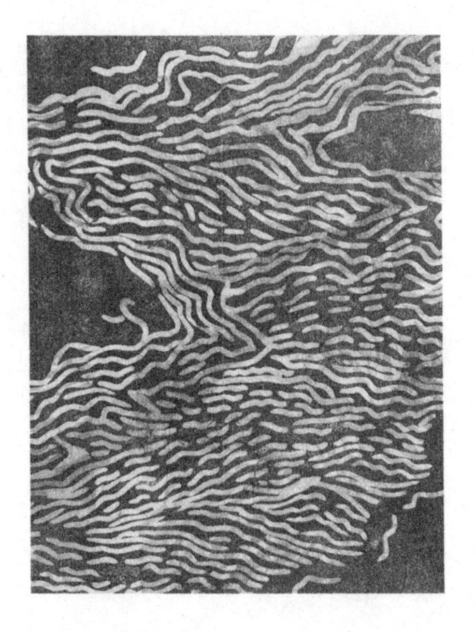

"No man steps in to the same river twice, for it's not the same river and he is not the same man" observed the Greek philosopher Heraclitus. You will get back in balance after loss and struggles, but your experiences have changed you and the world around you is always changing.

A conversation over tea

Green Tea Although I already suggested green tea in the Renourishing section, I want to invite you to drink some more because of the example it sets for a good approach to life. Artisan growers and processors (mostly in Asia) do not work with a set calendar in regard to harvesting tea leaves. They have learned when to prune the leaves and when to let them rest, accepting that this will be at different times according to climate, soil, and other factors. They work in harmony with Nature. You deserve to grow, develop, and rest on your own schedule. You need to grieve losses, take new steps, and move forward at your own pace, not one dictated by society or influential people in your life. Wow, I sure made green tea leaves into something very serious, but in much of Asia, tea growing, brewing, and drinking is serious business.

Plan to change

FIGURING OUT YOUR NEXT STEPS after trying to have a baby is far more difficult and complex than choosing the right foods, exercising more, or reducing exposure to unhealthy substances. My strategies below will, hopefully, help you recover your sense of identity, strength, and possibility to help you move ahead.

There's a good chance you will cycle through these changes several times in your lifetime and not just after trying to have a baby. Next steps may involve changing your career, priorities, and goals.

Life is a bit like a mobile made with weighted objects placed on horizontal rods that counterbalance each other. A gentle breeze or a slight touch sets them in motion, disturbing the appearance of balance. Circumstances throw us off balance, because life is neither static nor wholly predictable. But equilibrium always returns, because we are psychologically designed to seek and return to it.

You have suffered unfair loss and disappointment. But as psychologist Andrea Bonier points out, "Accepting that life is not fair doesn't mean giving up."[82] My intention in answering your questions up to this point has been to provide information that will help you re-establish your physical and emotional vitality as you make plans and take your next steps.

Now I want to share information and ideas on what your journey might look like going forward and answer questions about things that might temporarily shift the equilibrium in your emotional mobile.

I am not a psychologist specializing in fertility issues. I am a nurse-acupuncturist who has listened for more than 20 years to women who bravely kept putting one foot in front of the other each day as they faced fertility challenges. And I have noted what things seemed to help them move forward.

Neither I nor any therapist can tell you exactly what your next steps should be. You know in your heart what is best for you, and you wrote the owner's manual for you. However a close friend, or if necessary a good counselor, can help you reach into your heart for direction.

One of the things that I have observed in patients is that having a plan greatly reduces the kind of free-floating anxiety that comes with continually pondering the question of what your life will be like without a child or without more children. I phrased it, "without *more* children," because I have learned that the desire for a second or third child can be as intense as the desire for the first one.

---

82 Bonier, A., "Detox Your Thoughts: Quit Negative Self-Talk for Good and Discover the Life You've Always Wanted," *Chronicle Prism*, 2020

It was random that you had fertility challenges. I am not a believer in the "It was in God's plan" theories. The God I believe in wants you to multiply and does not want you to suffer. Having a plan removes the element of randomness from the rest of your journey and empowers you to move ahead instead of waiting for a plan from above to unfold.

In my theme of "Re" words—renourish, reinvigorate, reclaim, replenish—there is only one "re" word I want you to stay away from as you make your plans. That is "reliving." "What if I had eaten better? weighed less? been younger? or chosen a different doctor?" These are unhelpful and unanswerable questions. Try very hard to stay away from that interview with yourself. It will be like walking backwards.

I pretty much don't have a clue what my next steps will be. And just when I think I know, I change my mind. How can I possibly make any progress?

It may be frustrating, but it is common to be indecisive. Along with the importance of *having* a plan is embracing the thought that you have the right to *change* the plan at any time. In fact, it is common to change your mind when in treatment for fertility. A study about "decisional conflict" in couples in treatment for infertility discovered that "Changing decisions over time was another common theme . . . from one quarter to a third of couples changed their minds about how to proceed in family-building." Women's scores were higher than men's for "uncertainty about issues."[83]

83 Anguzu, A., Cusatis, R., Fergestrom, N., Cooper, A., Schoyer, KD., Davis, JB., Sandlow, J., Flynn, KE. "Decisional conflict among couples seeking specialty treatment for infertility in the USA: A longitudinal exploratory study," *Hum Reprod.* 2020 Mar; 35(3): 573–582.

I wrote this book for all of those who have decided they will be continuing to try to conceive, for those who have decided they will not, and for those who don't know yet. Moving between these categories is part of the journey. In addition to moving between categories, your need to Renourish and Revitalize will present at different times in your life in a cyclical pattern, not just in reproductive years. In that way, life is not a journey but a cycle, which is the Native American view of life. Those of us in the fertility field often refer to trying to have a baby as a journey, but a journey implies a distinct beginning and end, and you know it is not that simple. Needs once met resurface, emotions once dispatched are felt again, and challenges reoccur in our lives.

If you don't know whether you want to continue trying to conceive or to seek fertility treatments, clearly and unapologetically "own" this indecision. Then, make a plan for continuing to Renourish the spiritual and physical you until you *do* know. That way, you will be in the strongest possible place to act on your future plan. Renourishing is accomplished by the things I have written about in this book—eating well, staying physically strong, and never passing up an opportunity to grow spiritually.

If you really are in a quandary about what you want to happen at this point in your life, try this exercise. A friend learned this at a workshop a long time ago, so I don't know whom to credit for it. Get a piece of paper and a pen or pencil. Write ten sentences that begin with "I want." Write them quickly, one right after another, without pausing to ponder. This part is important. When you are finished, you may have at least some indication of what is important to you as you plan.

There is one thing I know you are not indecisive about because you have said this to me many times: "I just want to get back to my old self." You will accomplish the essence of that goal in time, but remember the words of the ancient Greek philosopher Heraclitus: "No person steps into the same river twice, for it is not the same river, and she is not the same person." The river keeps flowing. Your journey has formed and changed you.

Yes, I do just want to get back to my old self, but some days I just think, "Who was I, and who am I now?"

Let me tell you who you are not.

You are *not* an advanced maternal ager, a chronic miscarrier, a diminished ovarian reservist, or a poor responder. Recovering your identity begins with dropping these labels and the images they conjure up—not because the diagnoses were incorrect, but because so many women with these diagnoses are happy women and mothers. As you move forward, leave the medical labels behind.

I will always remember Ellen. She was 37 years old and came to acupuncture in preparation for the transfer of her last preserved embryo. She and her husband had decided this would be their last attempt at becoming parents. Although she had undergone surgery to remove extensive endometriosis, several IVF cycles had failed, and she was told that endometriosis was likely the reason. She came to her first appointment with a stack of color photos of her endometriosis taken during a laparoscopy. With downcast eyes, she presented them to me as if it were her calling card or portfolio. I gently told her that I did not want to look at the photos because I wanted to look at her, Ellen, the whole person, with all the necessary organs to conceive, and, just as importantly, the strong *will* to conceive. I suggested she throw the photos away and never look at them again. Happily, her embryo went to the trouble of splitting before it implanted, and she delivered healthy twin boys nine months after the transfer.

In 2017, the American Medical Association supported a resolution by the American Society of Reproductive Medicine to have infertility designated a disease. This is good because it may lead to better insurance coverage for fertility care. But try not to think of yourself as diseased. This is not a form of denial but is simply a way of reminding yourself that you are a whole person, not a diagnosis or a label. People with all sorts of diagnoses conceive and build their families. They were not necessarily "cured" of their disease or problem. They were healed, which literally means to be *made whole*. As a fertility patient named "Gabrielle" said in a February 2, 2009, *New York Times* article, "There really should be a word in between fertility and infertility." If you have all the parts, you are potentially fertile. Even if you have to borrow some parts to make a baby, your fertility cup is half full, not half empty.

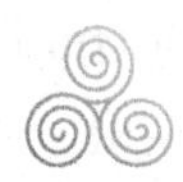

Relationship stuff. Same page, different paragraphs.

I think my next steps are to keep trying to get pregnant. My partner is conflicted about continuing to try. If we are not on the same page, won't that really stress our relationship?

As a bystander, this is what I have observed: A lot of couples are on the same page but not in the same paragraph.

They both want to start their family, but often the man has more financial concerns about family building—not because he does not want to spend money on trying to have a baby, but because he wants to be a good provider and be sure that there is money left for the start of a college fund. My intake form lists the question, "What is your reason for seeking acupuncture?" While a woman usually answers, "To help me conceive," a prospective father will often write, "To support my wife," or "To help my wife have a baby so she will be happier." A woman's strong maternal longings are baked in. In my experience, a woman is more likely to trust that everything will work out financially and that babies will be provided for somehow. But even my single patients have two voices inside them. One is saying, "I will be a great mother, no matter what; I have wanted a baby all my life," and the other voice is saying, "How, just how, will you afford college?"

My heart went out to my patient Heather when she came for treatment and shared that she had just been laid off from her pharmaceutical-sales job. She was due to start the stimulation phase of IVF the next day. It was obvious she had been crying. I assumed she was upset about her being laid off, but it turns out she was happy to have relief from the stress of getting to ultrasounds and blood draws while trying to work. She had been crying because, when she told her husband Dan about being laid off, he expressed concerns about moving forward with IVF due to the costs. "When we started IVF, we both had jobs," he reminded her. This observation landed him in deep doo-doo, as she viewed this as a lack of support. Like many partners, he wanted her to be happy, maybe even more than he wanted a child. Heather and Dan completed the IVF cycle with the help of marital counseling, where they learned to appreciate each other's emotions. Their IVF was successful; I'm sure that they have a better relationship and are better parents having learned that appreciation skill.

I don't know if my patients Natalia and Marco ever reached a point of appreciating each other's emotions. At our initial consult, a fertility app alarm on her phone went off. She announced to him that it signaled that she would be ovulating that night (no apps are that accurate) and that he needed to plan for that. He resented her unromantic approach, and they proceeded to have a scary, angry exchange right there in my office. I reached for the list of counselors that I keep on hand; fortunately there is a growing number who specialize in fertility issues.

Although "timed intercourse" (the euphemism for methodical sex near ovulation) is not that much fun, loving intimacy can and will return with attention to the emotional foreplay. By that, I mean being gentle, kind, and supportive outside as well as inside the bedroom.

If you are partnered, you are still two different people. Fertility will not be the only challenge in a long-term relationship, but it is definitely one that can strain a relationship. Conventional wisdom and marriage counselors would agree that expressing honest emotions is key to dealing with relationship issues. But candor is not always the best medicine. Saying everything that comes to mind can be hurtful and unproductive. Biting your tongue about minor transgressions or things that cannot be changed is not being dishonest—it is being kind. That's my best advice based on 45 years of marriage.

My partner has been there every step of the way for me. But I worry: Will this change if I want to do another round of IVF?
I am so happy to hear about the support you have. A relationship can be strengthened by the stress of infertility or miscarriage rather than weakened by it. Bones crumble unless we do exercises that put weight on them and stress them.

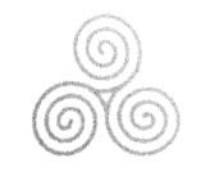

Dealing with the just-want-to-helpers

I am so tired of dealing with everybody's advice about what I should do next. If I keep trying to have a baby, or decide not to, how am I supposed to respond to intrusive questions about where I am in this process?

YOU HAVE LEARNED MANY THINGS about people during your time trying to conceive, including the tendency for family and friends to offer all sorts of suggestions about how to conceive or how to avoid another miscarriage. The pressure to take steps and make plans that involve what your parents or in-laws think you should do can be intense. I understand how this must feel, as I have had parents contact me to ask if I would call their adult child to tell them about my fertility practice. When I gently explain that it is not appropriate for me to do outreach, they always understand. When patients do begin treatment following a parent's recommendation, I sometimes get calls from them asking about progress. Thank goodness for HIPAA.

While you may not have always appreciated unsolicited suggestions, try to remind yourself that the people you love and who love you back are, indeed, just trying to help. Being grateful for compassionate family members who want you to be happy can help you heal. Advice offered in kindness may offer solutions to problems you have been struggling with. It is, however, perfectly fine to metaphorically plug your ears if the office shrew or an annoying neighbor asks questions that are none of their business.

"Do you have kids?" "Have you started trying yet?" I don't feel that these questions come from a place of kindness or compassion. Don't you think they just sound nosey?"

Yes. But interestingly, the people asking these questions, especially when they are not close friends or family, do not necessarily even care what the answers are. I remember being asked about whether I had children when I was young. When I stopped coloring my hair, it became, "Do you have grandchildren?" I often felt people simply wanted the opportunity to talk about their own grandchildren, as evidenced by the fact that, before I could even answer, they were pulling grandkid photos up on their phone. This tendency for people to ask you a question in order to talk about themselves gives you a tool to deflect questions by just turning the question back to them. "Do you have kids?" if they are reproductive age, or, "Do you have grandkids?" if they are older. They might not even notice you didn't answer their question.

It can also be helpful to have a mental inventory of stock responses. Think about the questions that bother you the most, and prepare your responses. One of my patients really hated being asked if she had tried IVF yet. Having to repeat that she had tried several times with no success just brought back a lot of sadness. An answer to the "Have you tried IVF yet?" question could be something soft, like, "We do, indeed, have a plan for starting our family." Or it could be something more direct, like, "That is private, between me and my partner," or "I don't like to discuss private medical information." The point is to have your responses you are comfortable with ready.

If you have suffered a miscarriage, you probably have been asked questions that you just don't feel like discussing on some days, like "How many weeks were you?" "Do the doctors know why you miscarried?" "Are you going to try again?" One of the best responses I have heard was from a dear friend who had two vibrant sons in their 20s, who died in tragic accidents within a few years of each other. When asked in social situations if they had children, she or her husband would simply respond, "We have two sons. They live in our hearts," without offering any additional information. People usually did not ask follow-up questions, which was the way the parents wanted it. Miscarriage commonly happens at six to eight weeks, but sometimes couples feel judged for grieving such an early loss. When people ask, "How far along were you?" you can say, "Our tiny baby left us early." Some people feel sad that no one asks them questions. This can be due to a lack of understanding regarding how devastating a miscarriage can be, or people may fear that questions will upset you. If it helps you to talk about your miscarriage rather than deflect questions, know that it is more than okay to do that. People may not always know the right words to use to comfort you, but that is, in part, because only you know the pain of your loss.

I wish there was a less clinical term for "chemical pregnancy," because I have often heard women sadly explain, "Yes, I got pregnant, but it was a chemical pregnancy," or "I was only a few weeks pregnant." It is as if they have sensed that women are not supposed to be sad about early losses, and so they are holding back. Let yourself be sad, and grieve about pregnancy loss at any stage.

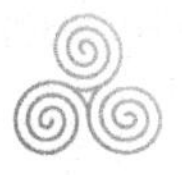

Calling Dr. Google

I never really understood why some people with my infertility diagnosis got pregnant, but I didn't. Before I decide if I am going to keep trying to have a baby, I'd like to get more information about my diagnosis and options. But the Internet seems like a black hole. How do I sort it all out?

HELPFUL AND AMAZING INFORMATION ABOUNDS on the Internet. But unhelpful and misleading information is also plentiful, and it can often be difficult to decipher which you have landed on.

Google is an amazing search engine, but you must remember that its brilliance is in helping you find websites and information, not in checking the legitimacy of the sites and accuracy of the information, and, even if reliable, whether it applies to you. I hate to see my patients spend large amounts of time searching for medical information, therapies, supplements, and doctors, only to become more confused. Take breaks from chronic search habits and Internet binges, and try to find a knowledgeable person (not just someone in a chat room) to talk to about things you discover—especially if it is a treatment or supplement you want to try during your next steps.

I advise going to academic medical sites designed for lay people, like MayoClinic.com, or ClevelandClinic.com and peer-reviewed medical journals like *Fertility and Sterility*. Medical journal articles can quickly get esoteric and detailed. The statistics course you took in grad school eight years ago will not prepare you for the mind-numbing pages of charts and graphs in many articles. Know that information from one positive study does not necessarily mean it can be applied clinically or that it proves that a treatment is safe and effective. Statistics can be interpreted differently, and it is well known that when studies are repeated, they rarely yield exactly the same results. The American Society for Reproductive Medicine (ASRM.org) has a good FAQ section, and FertilityIQ.com does a great job translating medical information from pertinent studies.

If you search for information on less academic and more consumer friendly sites, you should ask yourself this: "Do the claims about the therapy or intervention seem too good to be true?" or "Is this something my doctor has ever mentioned?" If you do read about something that resonates with you or that you are curious about, please don't be afraid to ask your doctor for fear of taking up their time or being judged. You should always check with them about supplements and treatments outside of mainstream medicine. Doctors are used to being asked about information patients find on the Internet, and they would rather have you ask than do or take something that might be harmful. Even though he or she may not be familiar with all products or therapies available (which is understandable), your doctor can offer an opinion about whether safety and efficacy bases are covered.

I pride myself on being open-minded, but I did put my foot down with Brin, who had suffered two miscarriages. Her sister gave her an electronic device she found online, *guaranteed* to help prevent miscarriage. It was a rubber pad that emitted some type of electricity that she was supposed to sit on every day for twenty minutes. I told her that, if she didn't send it back, I would come to her house and take it from her. I do have to admit, though, that my strong opinion was based on just one article I saw about a higher rate of miscarriage in women who sleep under electric blankets.

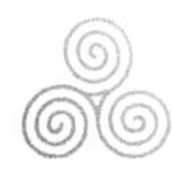

Witch doctors and which doctors

Should my next steps include chiropractic or Ayurvedic medicine for fertility? I also saw something called Mayan abdominal massage advertised at a wellness spa.

Rather than taking your time to go through every alternative therapy, I am going to make it easy for you and take the Marie Kondo "Less is More" approach to addressing complementary and alternative medicine, aka CAM.

Oh, and just so practitioners of complementary and alternative medicine don't send me nasty emails about implying CAM practitioners are witch doctors, you should all know that witch doctors were highly regarded throughout history and in many cultures for their ability to successfully treat ailments that mainstream doctors could not. Complementary and alternative medicine does not just refer to strategies that have roots in ancient history, like acupuncture and Ayurvedic medicine. People have thought up new uses for everything from lasers to blasts of cold air (cryotherapy) to help with what ails you, and this is now a part of CAM.

Most alternative and complementary strategies do not have much scientific or evidence-based research to conclusively prove that they help general or reproductive health. There is, however, abundant anecdotal evidence and many personal testimonials. I believe that some alternative and complementary strategies can help a person relax, which would dilate blood vessels and theoretically increase blood flow to organs. Better blood flow, better function of organs. Many patients have told me that yoga keeps them sane and that chiropractic has helped their musculoskeletal pain. This is good. Although I personally do not understand how manipulating someone's spine (as in chiropractic) can help them conceive or cure their ovarian cyst and hot flashes, I do not roll my eyes when a patient tells me about their positive experience. This is because for more than 20 years, I have inserted needles into specific points on the body, hoping to enhance hormone balance and fertility. Most people I see come for treatment after trying a lot of strategies, including multiple IUIs or IVFs. So when they have a course of acupuncture, and finally conceive (which has happened hundreds of times in my 20 years of practice), it both impresses and pleases me.

It is always a good idea to ask an alternative practitioner about his or her "success" rates and credentials. Don't get seduced by a well-designed website. Asking around and seeing which names keep coming up is important—but not just a "My sister-in-law's neighbor's cousin went to this guy who cured her hormonal headaches." You want direct testimonials from people standing in front of you.

Googling the name of a treatment modality followed by NIH.gov (National Institute of Health) or going to Google Scholar can take you to sites with academic research. But you won't find many clinical trials on homeopathy, essential oils, or chiropractic there. Try to read studies that are in peer-reviewed, scientific journals, not ones that are written by product manufacturers or a researcher not affiliated with an academic institution.

If you read about a treatment or search for information, Timothy Caulfield, author of *The Cure for Everything*, has some good advice, "Be skeptical, be scientific, be self-aware, be patient, and look for the best and most independent information."

Okay, I appreciate the answer about alternative stuff, but can I just ask you a quick question about essential oils? My sister was not having periods until she started using them. Does that sound possible?

As you may know, essential oils are concentrated, highly fragrant oils extracted from plants. They are usually diluted in "carrier" oils for massage, oil diffusers, or bath water. Some do indeed have therapeutic properties but can be harmful if not used properly.

While there is a lack of original research on the efficacy of essential oils, an article in the *Journal of Pediatrics* impressed me with the potentially powerful effects of essential oils. The author was a pediatrician in Denver who had two prepubescent boys as patients, unknown to each other, who were brought in by their mothers because they appeared to be growing breast buds. Careful history taking revealed that both boys had a foot fungus that their mothers were treating by lathering them with tea-tree oil, several times per day. There is good research to show that tea tree oil has anti-fungal and anti-bacterial properties. But the plant that it comes from, the *melaleuca alternifolia*, also contains phytoestrogens, which can mimic the effect of estrogens in the body. So, at pubescence, when body tissues are sensitive to hormonal stimulation, the boys were probably absorbing too much oil, which accounted for the breast buds.[84]

The paradox here is that essential oils may or may not help irregular periods or heavy menstrual flow but definitely have the potential to exert an action on the body.

If you are interested in trying essential oils, my friend Patty, who is an RN certified in essential oils, advises people to seek out high-quality, therapeutic-grade oils and get guidance from a certified aroma therapist.

As you plan for hormonal balance and health, please be cautious about herbs, supplements, lotions, or potions that are marketed as fertility aids. If you choose to take herbs, do not take them in combination with prescribed hormones. There are knowledgeable and credentialed herbalists, but, in my opinion, the research at their disposal can tell them about the safety of only some—but not all—of the possible combinations of herbs and pharmaceuticals.

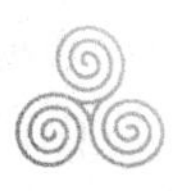

84 Korach, K., "Prepubertal Gynecomastia Linked to Lavender and Tea Tree Oils," *N Engl J Med* 2007; 356:479-485

Second opinions and reproductive "endocrinauts"

We really like our doctor, and her nurses are great about getting back to us and answering our questions. But we are not pregnant yet. If we decide to get a second opinion, how do we figure out which doctor would be best?

WHEN ASKED IF HE DID "SECOND OPINIONS," a very sought-after reproductive endocrinologist often replied to my patients, "I don't do second opinions. I do consults." I like that response, because, if you change doctors, you want a fresh look, not a critique or opinion about what any previous doctor could have done differently. There is no point to that. Your hormone levels, health status, age, and other factors may have been different when you were originally treated.

It is not uncommon for people to change doctors and clinics when trying to start their families. Patients have told me that, even though they really like their doctor, it feels illogical to repeat the same protocols and expect different outcomes. This logic does not always apply, because, for some people, it is just a matter of continuing to try to conceive that results in success, not a different dose of drugs.

I have seen my patients exhausted from trying to find the perfect fertility clinic, and then perhaps a second, third, or fourth. Many spend a ton of energy tracking down the latest Reproductive "Endocrinauts." I made up this last word as a fun way to refer to the docs who push the frontiers of reproductive medicine by adding tests and supplements to their protocols before there is enough research on efficacy to convince all of their peers to prescribe them. My made-up word was inspired by the Greek myth of Jason, who captained the ship *Argo* with a group of *nauts* (the Greek word for "sailor") and set out in uncharted waters to find the golden wool of Chrysomallos, a winged ram. Hence the words "astronaut" and "cosmonaut" came to mean intrepid explorers.

The British physicians Dr. Robert Steptoe and Dr. Robert Edwards bravely sailed on uncharted waters in 1978, when they performed the first successful IVF. Medical journals refused to publish their early results fearing fraud. Peers accused them of playing God. All they wanted to do was help women have babies. Working in a system of socialized medicine in post-World War II England, they did not seem to be seeking fame or fortune.

But the counterbalance to experimentation and progress is the use of protocols that are tried and true and do not put people at risk or compromise their health. It is fine to seek out a doctor who may specialize in your particular diagnosis, but I do not want you to ask yourself: "Should I have done IVF with Dr. A because she uses Viagra to thicken uterine linings?" or "Maybe I should see Dr. B because he recommends double the dose of vitamin D that I was taking, and he has women take DHEA." While some differences in these types of details could make a difference for some people, the big picture of fertility medications and procedures is standard. There are many excellent teams of fertility doctors that include both those who are happy if you eat well and take your pre-natal vitamins, and those who prescribe a long list of supplements.

Some of my patients choose a doctor based on the positive experience of a friend or chat group. Many of you have learned about the Society for Assisted Reproductive Technology (SART), the data bank to which doctors and clinics send their statistics on success rates for pregnancy and live births. It can be difficult to decipher direct comparisons between clinics, and the SART website itself states, "Accurate and complete reports of SART success rates is complicated. Clinics may have differences in patient selection, treatment approaches, and cycle-reporting practices that may inflate or lower pregnancy rates relative to another." If you really would like to understand clinic outcomes, I think the best approach is to ask the doctor you are considering to explain their clinic's relative success rates. If they can't, or won't, there may be a message there.

If your next steps involve changing your team of doctors, remember what you have told me over and over again: *Bedside manner matters.* A positive attitude on the part of the nurses and doctors, and good communication are vital. I don't mean that you should shop for a doctor who will "sugarcoat" the statistics on maternal age and chances of conception. But I do want you to find doctors and nurses who listen your goals and boost your confidence in your ability to conceive—by whatever means.

I have handed out a lot of Kleenex in my time as people described their first visit to a fertility doctor, when they perceived that the doctor was spending more time on statistics than listening to their goals. Kirsten expressed her strong desire to at least try to use her own eggs despite her advanced maternal age. The doctor tried to cheer her up by bringing out the egg-donor catalogue to show her a photo of a donor who, as he phrased it, "Looks just like you." He meant no harm and was trying to be positive. Doctors truly empathize when a patient expresses the pain of being behind schedule on having a baby, and, as healers, want to present the most expedient options for conception and relief from emotional pain. But Kirsten felt blindsided and did not get the opportunity to fully express her intense desire to use her own eggs. If you seek out multiple consults, be prepared for the fact that a doctor's approach may not be appreciably different from the other ones you have seen.

If you want to consult with another clinic, it is now easier than ever, due to the availability of teleconsults. Do plan to give yourself enough time to get your medical records transferred before your appointment, which can take time, even in this age of electronic records. Some of my patients are frustrated when a new specialist wants to repeat certain tests, but there are usually good reasons for repeating them. It is fine to ask what those reasons are.

If your next steps will include consulting with other teams, please don't exhaust yourself looking for the perfect clinic and team of doctors with exclusive access to all things reproductive. Having spent time, albeit vicariously, with dozens of fertility doctors in clinics all over the world (some of my patients have done IVF traveler.com), I can tell you that there isn't a perfect clinic, because people are not perfect. All clinics have positive and negative aspects and staff that you may click with—or not. Although various websites have testimonials and ratings of doctors, at some point, you have to evaluate the good care that you have already received—and then decide if making another change is in your best interests.

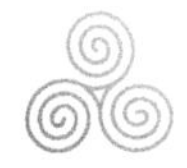

Natural family planning and frogs in shorts

I don't think finding a new doctor is going to help us. If this next IVF does not work, we are done—we're not doing another one. My fertility is probably age related, but my doctor said we could keep trying to conceive naturally. But that didn't work before—that's why we tried IVF. Should we even get our hopes up and try natural conception?

YES! AS I WILL MENTION AGAIN LATER, hope is, by nature, an emotion that exists against the odds. If you have all the parts, even if your sperm don't swim fast or you don't ovulate every month, you still have a chance.

Age-related fertility has been looked at mostly in the captive population of IVF patients, but the modest number of studies on natural conception and age have revealed some reasons for cautious optimism. **Except for age, the things that enhance fertility for both men and women are largely within your personal**

control: eating for good health (and a baby), reducing stress, not using marijuana or tobacco, avoiding exposure to endocrine disruptors (e.g., stop microwaving plastics), and having more frequent intercourse.

If a man and a woman in the 35 to 40 age group have intercourse at least two times per week and more often at ovulation time, their chances are higher than couples who have intercourse only once a week. If you are of normal weight as opposed to overweight, you increase your chances at any age. If you have had children before, you will have a shorter time to pregnancy than women who are trying for their first. A 40-year-old woman who is partnered with a 30-year old man will have better chances than two 40-year-olds, because a man's fertility declines with age, too, albeit at a slower rate.[85]

It seems to me that much of the time the responsibility for working on the lifestyle factors falls on to the woman. This is not the fault of men. A man's contribution to conception was not even verified until the 1770s, when an Italian Catholic priest, Lazaro Spallanzani, put waxed shorts on a group of male frogs to see if the fluid they were spreading onto females was the reason for tadpoles.[86] Of course, it was known that babies came from women, but scientists were puzzled about the exact role of men, since babies only *sometimes* followed sex. When it was speculated that males of the species may indeed plant some kind of seed, because Spallanzani's frogs without shorts made tadpoles and the guys in shorts did not, the scientists knew they were on to something.

---

85 Dunson, D., "Increased infertility with age in men and women," *Obstetrics & Gynecology*: January 2004. Volume 103, Issue 1, pp. 51-56

86 *Seeds of Life,* Edward Dolnick, Basic Books, New York, 2017

When Father Spallanzani looked at frog fluid under a microscope (invented by his contemporary Antoni von Leeuwenhoek), he thought that the sperm swimming around were parasites and it was the ejaculate itself that resulted in pregnancy. (See "Frogs in Shorts and Cosmic Eggs" in Notes). Our understanding of the male contribution to conception has moved ahead since then, but attention to the importance of good nutrition, lifestyle, and stress reduction in the male often falls into soft focus when there are fertility challenges.

If your next steps include trying again to conceive naturally, I recommend not wearing waxed shorts to bed. Kidding aside, consider getting treatment or a new consult for any male-factor diagnosis you may have received.

When undergoing IVF, low sperm count and low motility do not need to be addressed, because good-looking sperm will most likely be found in a semen sample when needed.

However, normal sperm count, motility, and shape (morphology) are associated with fertility as well as general health. Men can increase their chances of conceiving naturally if men do everything they can to support sperm health. Sperm are sensitive to heat, so to increase sperm counts, a potential father should avoid hot tubs, extreme bicycling, and using a computer on his lap.

Sometimes, when both the man and woman have a fertility challenge and proceed to IVF, the surgical correction of a "mechanical" reason for a low sperm count, such as correcting a varicocele is not pursued. Varicoceles are varicose veins in the testes that warm the sperm too much, which slows them down and impacts their longevity. If you will be trying to conceive naturally, consider visiting a urologist to see if a varicocele might be the reason for low sperm count and motility and if a repair might be an option. Varicoceles are common and do not necessarily require surgery, nor do they result in sterility, but from 30% to 50% of men who have the repair will go on to father children within a few years after repair. Simply continuing to try to conceive does, of course, factor into the success rates here.

If we try again on our own, what's the best way to track ovulation and time intercourse?

Let me share my views on ovulation prediction first. Then I will move on to advice on the most important and fun part of trying to start a family.

There are a lot of ways to determine when ovulation might occur, but there is no technology that is foolproof or can tell you the exact hour that ovulation will or did occur. Hours matter, since the egg lives only 12 to 24 hours and does best if approached by a sperm in its first 4 to 6 hours. Sperm can live up to 72 hours, but many are dead before then, so the "up to" is a bit misleading. The fertile window widens as they hang out in the fallopian tube waiting to meet an egg, so arriving before an egg is released is a good strategy. Sperm arrival time will vary and cannot be precisely known. It is amazing that *anyone* gets pregnant, given all the things that must be lined up, but they do. I know it is frustrating that, even with everything seemingly "lined up," pregnancy does not occur 80% of the time after sex in any given cycle. But I figured out why Mother Nature arranged it that way—you heard it here first. She had to make the "act" pleasurable, otherwise, no one would ever "do it." But can you imagine if every time couples copulated, a baby was born nine months later? I am thinking the planet would sink into the cosmos.

You have probably tried ovulation-predictor kits, which measure the luteinizing hormone responsible for stimulating an egg to grow. The amount of time from a detectable level of LH until an egg is released is estimated to be about 24 to 36 hours. Based on the thousands of sticks peed on by my patients, it appears that sometimes they ovulate *after* they get a positive test, and sometimes they don't. Or they ovulated (as evidenced by conception) and never "caught" a positive result. One of my patients is a mother of four and never *once* got a positive home LH test result for any of her four pregnancies. Do careful research on other products that claim to predict ovulation, like bracelets and vaginal monitors. I am not convinced the manufacturer's research proves accuracy.

You have probably heard about or tried temperature charting, which is based on the fact that most women will get a slight (around 0.5 degree) rise in their early morning (basal body) temperature after they ovulate. This is an accurate tool, but your technique must be flawless, including no or minimal movement upon waking and taking your temperature at the same time each morning. Most of my patients tell me that logging temperatures is annoying and stresses them. Because the temperature rises after an egg is released, it is not really a good method of ovulation prediction for any given cycle. However, if you have regular cycles, you can see when you might ovulate in subsequent months.

I actually didn't mind doing the temps. At least I could see that I was probably ovulating each month.

Yep, that is definitely a benefit. This is why I recommend that women who are wondering whether they are ovulating take early-morning temps, even for just a few cycles. The phone "apps" for predicting cycles are based on how many days previous cycles were and when you probably ovulated in those cycles. The catch here is that apps cannot factor in things like illness, stress, and other unknowns (the moon?) that can shift the phases of a cycle.

Comprehensive natural family planning involves paying attention to signs of impending ovulation like the appearance and characteristics of cervical mucus. It is clear, shiny, slippery, looks like uncooked egg white and does not necessarily stretch to the length you see in on-line images. It is not watery, yellow, white, or sticky, which cervical mucus is at other times in the cycle. Putting this fertile mucus together with bloating, skin blemishes, light cramping, or other things you associate with ovulation is key to best timing for intercourse. Body signs (other than mucus) can be non-existent or due to other causes, so testing your urine for luteinizing hormone can be helpful. Fertile mucus dries up after ovulation (probably the result of the progesterone coming out of the follicle that has now become a corpus luteum gland), so you may catch only a swipe of slippery, clear fluid on toilet tissue once during impending ovulation.

Don't worry if you don't detect fertile mucus flowing down through your vagina. Part of its job may be to hang out at the cervix to meet and greet the sperm and rehydrate them for the rest of their journey up to the tubes. As I mentioned earlier, many of my patients report that they never get this "fertile mucus" and view it as evidence that they are broken. But many of these same women are happy mothers now, so noticing its appearance is not a requirement for conceiving.

I have read so many different recommendations on when and how often to have intercourse. Every day around ovulation time, or every other day?
I have a good recipe that has led to success for many of my patients: have intercourse often.

* Have intercourse two to three times per week through your whole cycle and add a few more times during your mid-cycle. It is not necessary to have intercourse during heavy menstrual flow if you are not comfortable with that, but know that it is possible to conceive while still having a light flow.

* Then, if you get fertile mucus and/or an LH surge, have intercourse for three days in a row.

* You must continue having intercourse beyond the three days if you still have noticeable clear, slippery mucus, because that means you have likely not yet ovulated.

* I also recommend having intercourse at least one more time after the fertile mucus seems to have disappeared to "seal the deal." I mention intercourse two to three times a week to avoid having to focus so diligently on the "fertile window."

* Don't worry about depleting the sperm supply—the average man makes 1,500 sperm per minute. Good research indicates that, if you are around age 40, intercourse four times per week will increase the chance of conceiving. If this frequency is not possible in any given month, remember that even a "one and

done" approach can result in conception if the timing is right. Don't lose heart, and take a relaxed approach when you need to.

Busy lives and stress can make finding time for intercourse a challenge and decrease your desire for intimacy. I often think that it would be so much better if humans were like some mammals known as "ovulation induction" species. Female camels and llamas for example, do not even ovulate until they have intercourse with a male. Very economical. The existence of ovulation induction following exposure to seminal fluids in certain animals has been known by scientists for a long time, and they are still trying to figure out the "secret" ingredient that triggers the female to ovulate.[87] They have even discovered that seminal fluids with no sperm in them will stimulate ovulation.[88]

The effect on ovulation from exposure to seminal fluids is now being studied in humans.[89]

But I think the "secret" may be hiding in plain sight. Ejaculate is only 2% to 4% sperm, with the rest containing fluids from the prostate and a healthy dose of testosterone, estrogen, and progesterone. What a nice, symbiotic way Mother Nature created for a female to receive the estrogen she may need to mature an egg and the progesterone she needs to grow a nice uterine lining. When I asked a patient, who is a veterinarian, about ovulation induction, she added that cats are an ovulation-induction species as well. I said, "Uh, no—I think you

---

87 Underwood, E, "Semen's Secret Ingredient," https://www.sciencemag.org/news/2012/08/semens-secret-ingredient

88 Allali, K., "Effect of the Camelid's Seminal Plasma Ovulation-Inducing Factor/β-NGF: A Kisspeptin Target Hypothesis," *Front Vet Sci*, 2017, 4:99

89 Schjenken, J., "The Female Response to Seminal Fluid," *Physiol Reviews*, July 2020. P. 1077-1117

missed class on cat day at vet school." Female cats screech and go into heat and find a male if they can, and then have kittens. She explained that cats are hybrids, can get pregnant with a litter in the usual way, and then impregnated again at the same time if she was triggered to release more eggs after going on a date with a tomcat while pregnant. This occurrence is confirmed by seeing two litters of different ages on ultrasound. I know this information is interesting but not necessarily of use to you (since you are not a llama or a cat), unless you take a leap with me and believe that perhaps the extra hormones a woman absorbs from semen can be helpful for fertility. The takeaway here is that intercourse at all times of a cycle may *theoretically* coax an egg to mature or a lining to thicken. Interestingly, scientist and anthropologist Jared Diamond was told by indigenous people in New Guinea that intercourse right up until delivery time is common, "because they believe that repeated infusions of semen furnish the material to build the fetus's body."[90]

With kids and jobs, frequent intercourse can be a challenge. So, if you need to plan for it, don't get overwhelmed by using too many ways to track ovulation. Paying attention to body signs and glancing at your calendar to know when mid-cycle is coming are strategies that work well. If you are not regular, try LH-surge testing. Be practical—don't plan dinner parties during mid-cycle. You need to go to bed early instead of spending time cleaning up the kitchen.

90 Dolnick, E., *The Seeds of Life: From Aristotle to da Vinci, from Sharks' Teeth to Frogs' Pants, the Long and Strange Quest to Discover Where Babies Come From*, 2017, Basic Books, New York, p. 33

The emotions that will follow in your footsteps

PLANNING YOUR NEXT STEPS involves refocusing thoughts and realigning plans. You can feel like you are doing a good job at this, and then a wave of grief or sadness washes over you as you think about the baby you did not conceive. Or the one that "passed back into God's pocket," as my father used to say. You are not back to square one when this happens. It is normal for grief and sadness to ebb and flow, and to follow you at times as you take your next steps.

Do you mean I am always going to feel sad or angry when I go to baby showers? And if I keep having sad spells, could that interfere with getting pregnant in the future?
Grieving is not linear, meaning you do not necessarily feel a little better each day until finally you don't feel any sadness about your

loss. Grieving usually goes like this: You feel good one day, and you have not cried silently or outwardly. But then, the next day, you are a mess. Then more days pass, and they are all good, and you feel optimistic. And then the next day, like an unexpected wave hitting you as you stand with your back to the ocean, grief washes over you. As time goes on, the waves will be fewer, softer, and the intervals longer. There are many helpful books about how to deal with grief, but my personal belief is that you will always feel a sense of longing and curiosity about the baby that could have been yours. Whether your baby lived in your heart or spent time in your womb, the sadness, longing, and curiosity about him or her will occupy a smaller and smaller place in your heart as time goes by. You will take these emotions out and look at them at times, and then put them back as your busy and fulfilling life calls to you.

Many of my patients go on to have successful pregnancies within a few cycles after a miscarriage, at a time when they are still sad about a pregnancy loss.

Everyone will respond differently to fertility challenges. For some, grief and sadness may result in things like low libido, low energy, drinking too much, and inattention to nutrition, all of which will block the path to refocusing and healing. So if your grief does not seem to be moving toward resolution, or if you truly feel little joy in life, consider looking for a therapist skilled in grief counseling and knowledgeable about fertility struggles. I am impressed with the number of counselors now specializing in these issues.

Ideally, get a personal testimonial about someone you are considering seeing. My patient Kim went to a psychologist she found on the Internet whose website touted her skill working with patients going through IVF. As it turned out, three patients reported back that all she did was talk about her own miscarriage and subsequent successful IVF. While it can be reassuring that a counselor knows what you have been through, oversharing by this therapist was really not well received. I put this therapist on my *Dr. Not-to-call* list.

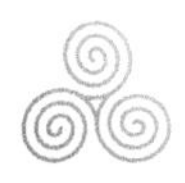

Fear, faith, hope, and happiness

YOU HAVE FELT GRIEF, SADNESS, ANGER, FRUSTRATION, disappointment, jealousy, and fear while trying to start a family. Some of these emotions will be with you for a while as you heal and plan your next steps. Grief and sadness can abate with time. Anger is "a map . . . meant to be respected, that shows us what our boundaries are . . . and where we want to go."[91] Frustration and disappointment are held at bay by practicing gratitude, an important survival skill. Jealousy is so useless that it will go away on its own if you learn to ignore it and refuse to feed it.

But fear can be the emotion that will hold you back the most from deciding on and taking your next steps. Many of my patients have told me about the deep, heart-piercing fear that they experience when they think about never having a child or more than one child. It is normal to fear growing old without the company

91 Julia Cameron, *The Artist's Way: A Spiritual Path to Higher Creativity*. Putnam, 2002

of adult children or the enjoyment of grandchildren. But this fear can gnaw at your capacity to live a joyful life.

So, how do you make fear go away?

The short answer is, "You don't, and you can't." We are programmed to hang on to fear, because it serves to protect us from risky situations.

The long answer came to me as I was talking with a cop on Michigan Avenue in Chicago. He was one of a dozen or so mounted police weaving in and out of traffic on Black Friday, the busiest shopping day of the year on Michigan Avenue. At one point, he was riding his chestnut horse against the flow of heavy traffic between two narrow lanes. The sides of the cars were almost touching the horse. Horns were honking, engines were groaning, buses were sneezing, and pedestrians were darting in between cars. At one point, the horse's ears lay back, and he seemed to freeze, but within a second he continued on between the cars. I am hardly an expert on horses, but the ones I rode years ago would spook and throw you off at a lot less commotion than what was happening on Michigan Avenue. I later approached the officer when I noticed that he and his horse had stopped at an intersection. I asked him how he teaches the horses not to be afraid. He said, "You don't. You can't. It's their nature to be afraid, and you can't change that." He went on to explain that you teach the horses to go forward even while they are afraid. He added that teaching them to go forward despite fear is a lesson that is never done. The horses must go out every day to stay in shape for the noise and traffic. I don't believe you must "conquer" your fear about the future or assume you need fear to go away as you step out into the emotional traffic of life.

Faith is an emotion that will help you move through fear—faith that your future will be fulfilling and meaningful, which, unlike conception, is something you can largely control. You can choose to keep growing and exploring, to help others and the Earth.

Embracing hope as you heal and plan your next steps will be like emotional fertilizer. There was a time when I felt as if I were selling false hope when I encouraged couples to keep trying to conceive naturally when their "numbers" were not ideal and their diagnoses complicated. I once had a patient who had only one ovary, and one tube inconveniently located on opposite sides of her uterus. She conceived naturally and birthed a healthy baby boy. Another memorable patient was born with two complete uteruses (not just a septum within one uterus), each with a tube and ovary; she was advised to have one of them removed. She was fearful of the procedure and just kept trying to conceive naturally. Which she did. Having seen so many beautiful babies born to couples with fertility challenges, I realized that there is no such thing as false hope. The very nature of hope is that it exists against the odds. Never let anyone take hope away from you with statistics, data, or inconsiderate comments.

I think I could make peace with not having children and not be afraid of being childless if I just knew what my future would be like. Will I eventually have a baby?

I like what Pope Francis had to say about living with things that cannot be known. He said it is like driving at night when you can see only as far as your headlights, but continuing to drive gets you there. Focusing on what is in front of you each day will coax you along the road to peace and happiness.

Yes, children bring happiness, but not having them does not doom you to a life of unhappiness. Researchers have tried to answer the question of whether parents are happier than non-parents; it seems like the answer should be straightforward, but it is not. So many factors come into play, such as whether having children was a choice, that it is difficult to arrive at a consensus. Part of the bottom line seems to be that there is a cost-benefit ratio when one is a parent *and* a cost-benefit ratio when one is *not*. And when I say "cost" in the context of parenthood, I mean things like the never-ending tendency for a parent to feel their child's pain even when they are adults, to disagree with their life choices, to become estranged from them or to lose them to premature death. Parenthood is worth these risks, but if these things happen, unhappiness will follow.

Children are neither a cure for depression nor a guarantee of well-being. I say that based on the fact that many of my patients were on antidepressants long before trying to start a family and remain on them after having children.

The benefits of not devoting your life to parenting probably do not seem appealing right now, so I won't get presumptuously preachy. But I am continually impressed with my former patients who have shared the joys of their travels, professional pursuits, and enriched extended family relationships that have come their way as they live their lives as non-parents or with fewer children than they wanted. I don't make them fill out a happiness questionnaire, but they truly seem happy and so much less stressed than when they were struggling to conceive.

Dina and Michael were several years and three IVFs into their journey when additional genetic testing revealed that Michael carried a gene that would make it nearly impossible for them to have a healthy baby. They have made concerted efforts to meet other couples who are not planning to have children, and having these new friends has really helped them feel positive about non-parenthood. Dina felt a sense of relief at not being distracted from life by the ticking of her biological time clock.

This whole conversation—and your whole journey—started because you wanted to have the happiness a baby can bring. The authors of our Constitution promised us Life, Liberty, and the *pursuit* of Happiness. They knew better than to offer a guarantee of happiness and were wise to imply it is something we need to put some effort into by pursuing it.

Please choose happiness when and where you see it. Better yet, make it happen by doing things that create it. Studies of multi-million-dollar lottery winners reveal that it is not being able to buy things that makes them happy. It is being able to do things and have new experiences that is the major contributing factor to happiness. You can do things and have new experiences without a lot of money and without children.

If you step back into the baby-making lane, which I hope you feel better prepared for after our conversation, you know that it will still be difficult and consuming. Please don't neglect the pursuit of happiness during that time. Along with having children, happiness is a great goal, and you deserve to have it.

With your fear, faith, hope and happiness inside you, I wish you all the best on the rest of this journey and cycle we call life.

God Bless,
Jane

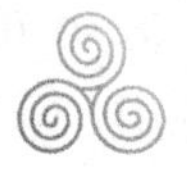

Notes

How to brew tea

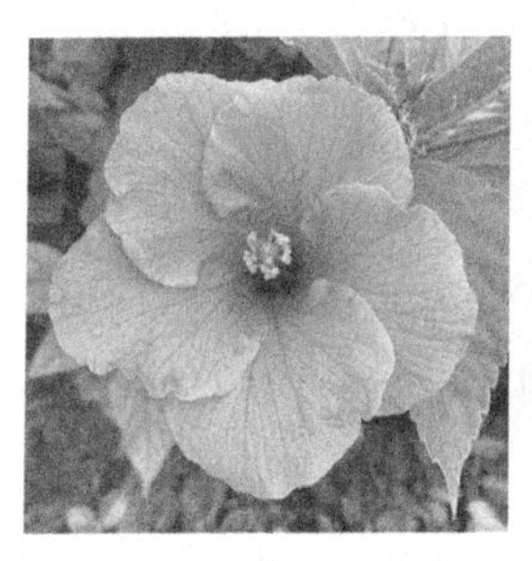
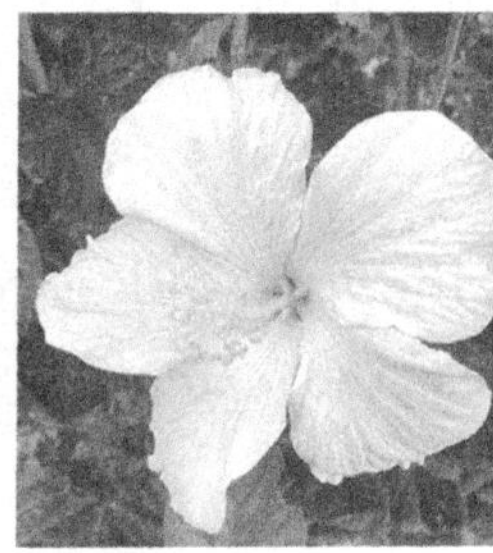
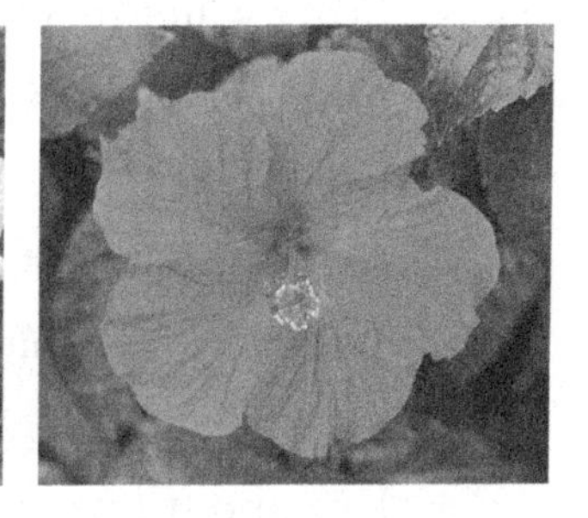

Hibiscus flowers come in pink and yellow, but it is the red ones that are used for tea.

Serious steeping

I learned about brewing at a tea school in China during my internship, and at a tea ceremony in Japan. Basically, serious steeping involves matching the type of tea leaf (black, green, herbal, etc.) with the ideal container (metal, glass, ceramic), heating water to specific temperatures for the type of tea, and then steeping it for a specific amount of time that is different for each tea. Detailed instructions on these variables can be found online.

Seriously steeping tea does indeed make a difference in flavor. I was never able to duplicate the tea I enjoyed in Asia because brewing tea is an art that people learn in special schools and learn from family.

Casual steeping

* This applies to loose tea or tea bags.
* Bring water to a full boil, but then let it cool for 30 seconds or so.
* Do not microwave the water unless you don't have options. Boiling "oxygenates" the water, and this is good.
* Use about one teaspoon of loose tea or one bag for six to eight ounces of water.
* Steep for the amount of time that results in the best flavor for you.
* Do not squeeze the tea bag after steeping unless you like your tea bitter.

Drink organic tea when possible. Non-organic has probably been sprayed a lot.

Enjoy in a glass or ceramic cup to avoid plastic chemicals.

Mindful breathing instructions

SIT OR LIE IN A COMFORTABLE POSITION, with your eyes closed or in "soft focus." (Taking your glasses off can help with soft focus.)

* Breathe in through the nose and out through the nose.
* Focus on the sound of the breath if you can hear one.
* Focus on the feel of the breath in the nose if you can feel it.
* You can visualize your breath entering and leaving your lungs if that keeps you focused on the breath.
* When thoughts come into your mind, observe what they are, let them go, and go back to the breath.

Remember that the mind was designed to think thoughts, just as your heart was designed to beat and your lungs to breathe. They do this automatically. You cannot stop your heart from beating just because you want to. So it is with the mind—its job is to think thoughts, and it will not stop simply because you want it to. Meditation is not about clearing your mind, which is not possible. It is about giving your mind one thought—the breath and the present moment.

If you have difficulty staying with the breath, try taking in a breath, and saying "one" as you exhale. Take the next inhalation and say "two" as you exhale. Only count to ten or so, and then start over at "one." I don't want you lying there saying to yourself, "Two thousand five hundred and seventy one . . ."

Begin by meditating at least 10 minutes per day. Work up to 20 minutes or more on your own schedule. It helps to have a regular time of day that you meditate, such as the first thing in the morning or just before bedtime.

Acupressure for calming your spirit

Yongquan (Chinese for Rushing Water) is the name of an acupuncture point on the bottom of the foot that is used to reduce "Uprising Yang" which can be manifested by agitation, insomnia, and a tendency to be fearful. It is located on the bottom of the foot, about 1/3 of the way down the foot from the base of the toes, in between the second and third toe. Kind of right below what you might think of as the fleshy ball of the foot. Use your finger or knuckles or a massage tool to apply firm pressure to the area, using the following pattern: 15 slow counts on the point, 15 slow counts off. Repeat sequence for about 3 to 5 minutes. Can be done daily.

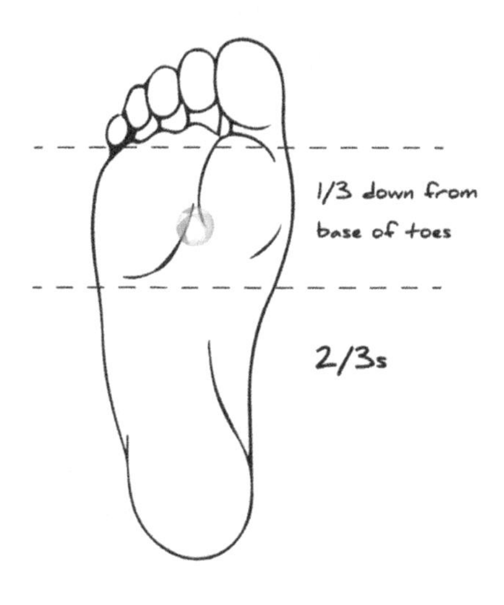

Repeat this pattern for about five minutes. There is nothing magical about the number of counts or times the pattern is repeated. The point is that it is not a constant pressure. Acupressure can be as effective as acupuncture in many situations and is the preferred method in *Yangquan* (called "Kidney 1" in English) for many people. You can do both feet at the same time or rotate, as often as you would like. There is a saying in ancient Chinese medical books, "Treat *Yongquan* every day, live for 100 years."

Links to good teachers of *Tai Qi* and *Qi Gong* classes

Kathy Lang. Her website has links to *Tai Qi* and *Qi Gong* online classes. She is calming and easy to understand. https://tcmtime.com/classes/

Helen Liang. She does not have her own website, but, if you access this one, you will find links to streamed classes and reasonably priced DVDs. Her classes are great for beginners. .https://ymaa.com/publishing/dvd/tai-chi-women

She can be found on YouTube at https://www.youtube.com/watch?v=apIffYvzuS0&ab_channel=STORYHIVE

Kseny. Her *Qi Gong* classes can be found on YouTube. https://www.youtube.com/channel/UCJYjsMmSjHqb4PhiUdCyRsg

Mimi Kuo-Deemer. She offers live-streamed *Qi Gong* classes and DVD options. Skilled and relatable teacher—website: https://www.mkdeemer.com/classes.htmlyoutube.com/channel/UCBtGM4p9zYXzu0bIlfvUJ9A

Refreshing resources

Environmental Working Group: www.ewg.org/ Most comprehensive source for safe product information, including food, cleaning products, and cosmetics. Great updates on pending environmental legislation in various states.

Because Health: www.becausehealth.org/ Tips and guidelines for safer cookware and non-toxic personal-care products.

Silent Spring Institute: www.silentspring.org/ Organization dedicated to researching the cause-and-effect relationship between environmental chemicals and health. They developed a free mobile app to help consumers get information on products and assess possible sources of contamination (silentspring.org/project/detox-me-mobile-app).

Made Safe: www.madesafe.org. Program that checks products for bad chemicals and "certifies" safe ones. Includes lists of cosmetics, personal-care items, cleaning products, bedding, and clothing.

Program on Reproductive Health and the Environment: www.prhe.ucsf.edu/ Their mission is to educate people who want to start a family about possible sources of endocrine disruption. Based at UCLA.

If you want to get involved and be proactive . . .

Clean Water Action: www.cleanwateraction.org This is a grassroots advocacy group that safeguards public health by working to support legislation that is environmentally important.

Earth Justice www.earthjustice.org Since 1971, their 160 lawyers have helped communities with legal problems related to toxic exposure and policies that harm the environment. If you become a client, their services are free.

The Union of Concerned Scientists www.ucsusa.org Scientific and research-based group that tries to foster responsible government policies and promote consumer-friendly corporate behavior.

If you would like to get involved in a local rather than national organization, many states and cities often have non-profit organizations dedicated to clean air and water at the local level.

Frogs in Shorts

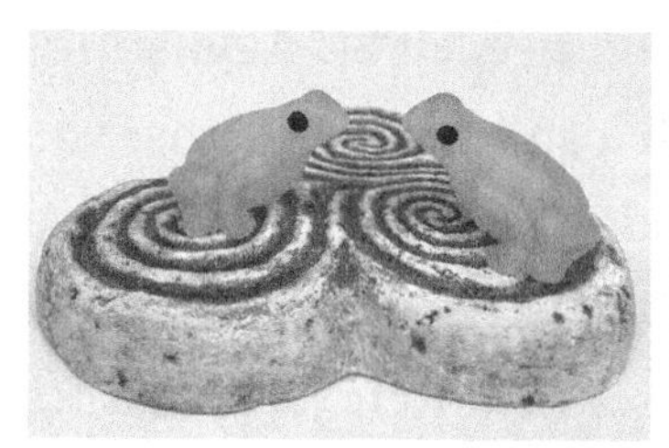
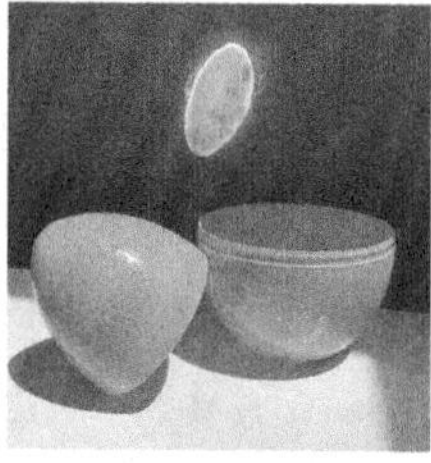
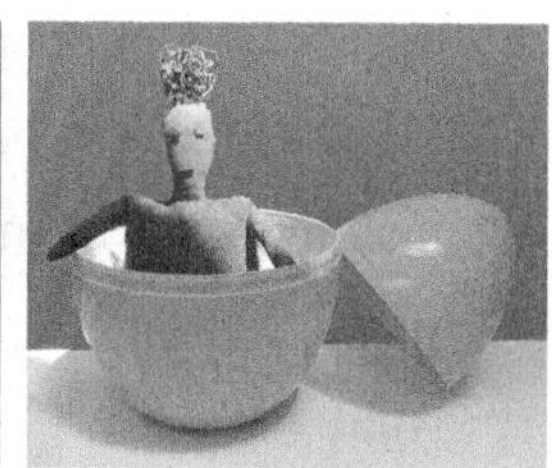

JUST LIKE YOU, Father Spallanzani had good questions about reproduction. His experiments in the 1760s documented the male contribution to reproduction by showing that male frogs in waxed shorts could not impregnate females. But he and contemporary Anton Leeuwenhoek (inventor of the microscope) agreed that the tiny wiggling things they saw were just parasites who swam around for a while in the male fluids and then died. They believed that the ejaculate itself was what resulted in pregnancy and that women were just fertile fields or incubators, with no contribution of their own. Many years later, scientists (known as spermists) agreed that sperm was definitely a player, and opposed the "ovists" who believed that women were the source of human reproduction and the ejaculate was just a trigger. Spermists believed that there was a fully formed human (homunculus) inside the sperm.

Ovists maintained that a little fully formed human was already inside a woman and was stimulated to grow by intercourse or the fluids. It was, of course, more difficult to prove a woman's contribution, due to the internal location of ovaries and eggs. Chickens were observed coming out of eggs, but birds and frogs were not seen as having common reproductive ground with humans. There were however, extreme ovists who believed that all of nature, including the entire planet, hatched from a giant cosmic egg. From 1600 to 1900, knowledge accumulated slowly, as people clung to Biblical quotes about "men planting seeds" and heeded St. Augustine's proclamation that body curiosity was a sin. By 1827, Ernst von Baer observed a mammalian ovum and put forth the theory that all mammals came from ovum. Interestingly, he, too, believed that spermatozoa (literally "animals of the semen") were just parasites in the ejaculate. Decades later, the ovists and spermists shook hands and agreed that a cell from a female mammal and one from the male, met, merged, repeatedly divided, and became an embryo.

There was still a bit of a thorny issue back then that, interestingly, remains with us today. When sperm and egg meet, merge, multiply, and become an embryo, what sets that in motion? A *spark of life*, a *vital force*, the *hand of God*? A spiritual or religious viewpoint would support the latter explanation. Some scientists and non-scientists believe the process of conception and life is chemistry, ruled by blind laws of nature. The question of why seemingly healthy ova are not always fertilized by willing sperm at every opportunity is one that both sides are pondering.

Made in United States
North Haven, CT
28 November 2023

44709599R00157